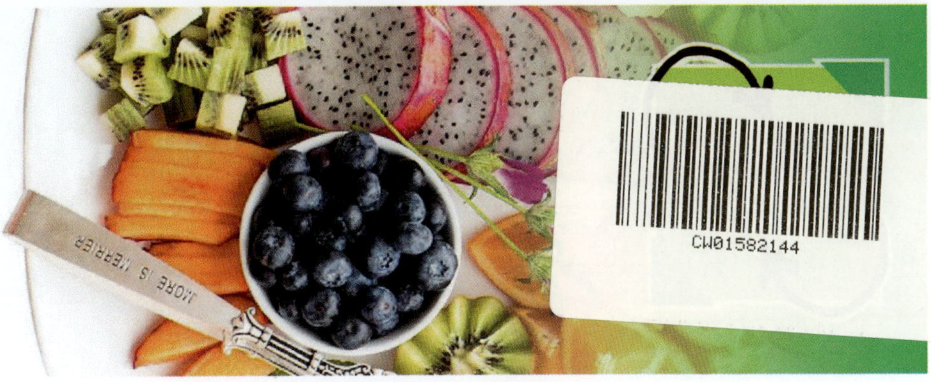

Exercise and Carb Cycling

OK so as mentioned on high carb day, exercise is best done on high and moderate days.

However, this does not require hours of work in the gym! The most effective type of exercise to pair with carb cycling, is a short HIIT session, just 10 to 15 minutes is perfect.

This not only gets your heart rate up, but actually keeps it going for longer, even more effective than a long run or an hour of strenuous activity. What's more, its so easy to do at home!

YouTube has an abundance of great videos, Just search for 15 minute HIIT and you'll be spoilt for choice!

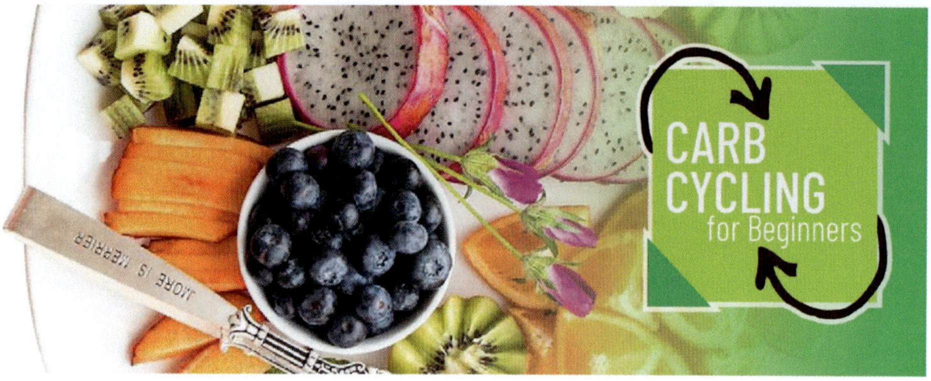

Eating Out

THIS can seem like a terrifying prospect when you are first starting out.

What will everyone else say when I order something different? How will I know what to order? How can I be sure what the restaurant will add to the food?

Luckily, the world has become better educated when it comes to low carb eating, and establishments - especially in the US - Are much more accommodating now to some odd requests.

I always say, keep it simple. For a low carb day, go for grilled meats; steak, chicken, pork chop, with sides of salads and vegetables, and you can even have a cream-based sauce to go with it. In the Indian restaurants have a curry - ask for some spiced veggies as an accompaniment and a creamy raita dip.

At the Italian, salads are the best way to go on low carb days; Caprese, Caesar, Goats cheese.

For high carb days you can have pasta! But only with a tomato-based sauce, Arrabiatta is a perfect choice. Gyro's are great but be sure it has a low fat dressing!

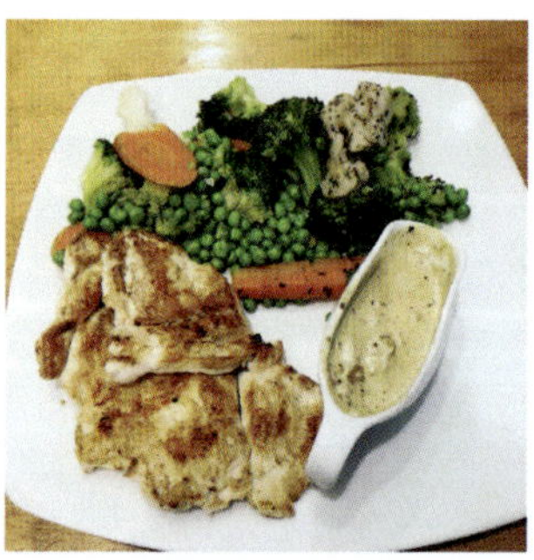

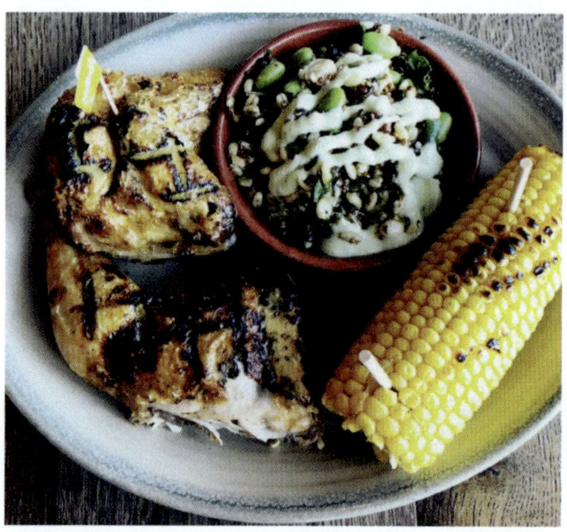

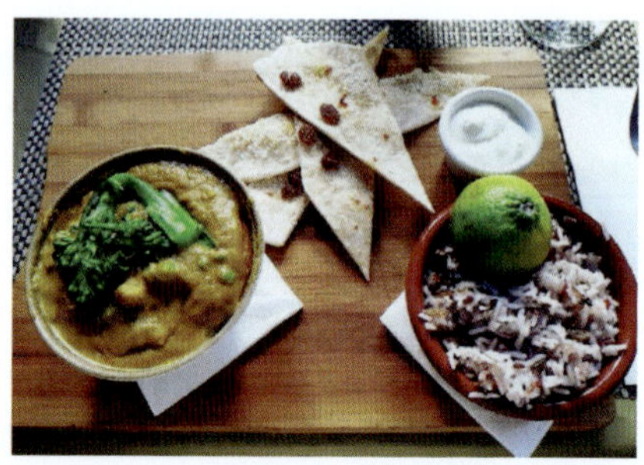

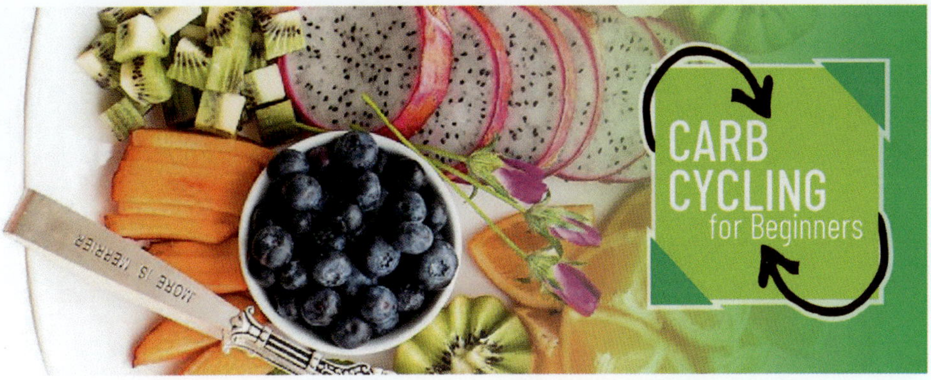

The Science Behind Carb Cycling

The science is primarily based on the biological mechanisms behind carbohydrate manipulation. Carb cycling tries to match the body's need for calories or glucose. For example, it provides carbohydrates around the workout or on intense training days.

The high-carb days are also in place to refuel muscle glycogen, which may improve performance and reduce muscle breakdown. Strategic high-carb periods may also improve the function of the weight- and appetite-regulating hormones leptin and ghrelin. The low-carb days are reported to switch the body over to a predominantly fat-based energy system, which may improve metabolic flexibility and the body's ability to burn **fat as fuel** in the long-term.

Another big component of carb cycling is the manipulation of insulin. The low-carb days and targeting of carbs around the workout may improve insulin sensitivity, a vital marker of health. In theory, this approach will maximize the benefits carbohydrates provide.

BOTTOM LINE: The proposed mechanism of carb cycling is to maximize the benefits of carbohydrates and teach the body to burn fat as fuel.

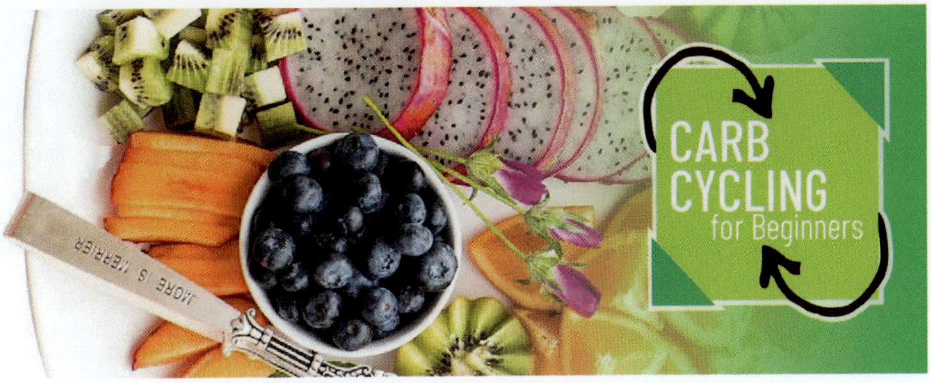

Does Carb Cycling Have Any Other Benefits?

As already mentioned, carb cycling has the potential to provide some benefits that other diets cannot. By having periods of low and high-carb, you may get many of the benefits provided by both diets, without some of the negatives.

Benefits of low-carb periods may include better insulin sensitivity, increased fat burning, improved cholesterol and enhanced metabolic health. High-carb refeeds may also have positive effects on hormones during a diet, including thyroid hormones, testosterone and leptin.

These factors may play an important role in long-term dieting success, since hormones play a key role in hunger, metabolism and exercise performance.

BOTTOM LINE: Low-carb periods may provide a number of health benefits, and high-carb refeeds can have positive effects on your hormones.

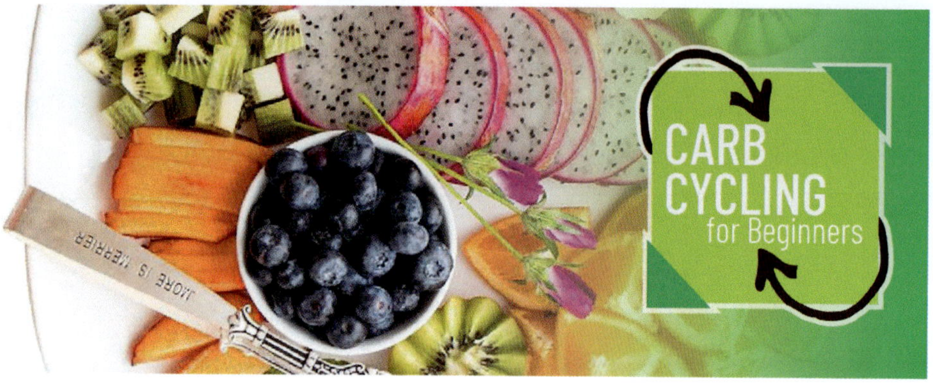

How Do I Carb Cycle?

THE question I possibly get asked the most.

There is no 'one size fits all' approach, as we all have different weights, ages, fitness levels and daily routines. Part of my program contains the crucial part – **Calculating Macros.**

Once you know how many grams you can eat of carbs, protein and fat, then here is your starting point.

The only thing which stays consistent is that on low carb days everyone has a limit of 50g carbs, whatever your weight.

The recommended cycle is Low, Low, Moderate, High and repeat.
Because of the exercise limitations, many people tweak this to suit their own fitness regime. For example I always save a high carb day for a weekend!

I recommend a good app to track your macros even if you have my meal plan, which makes it easier to check substitutes or any spontaneous snacks!

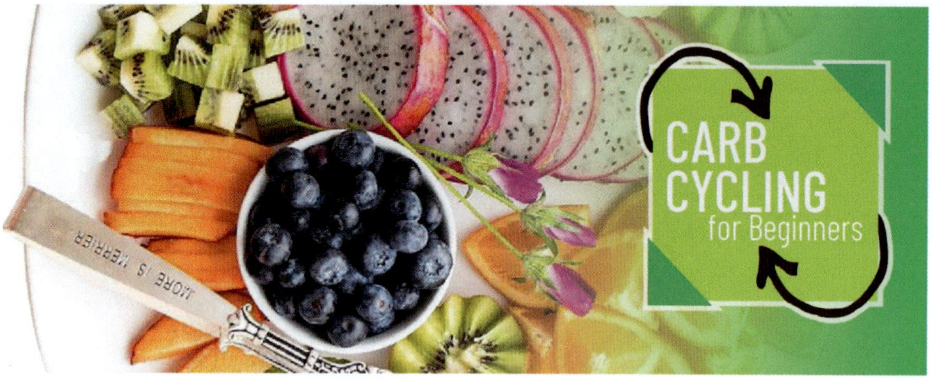

Can Carb Cycling Help You Lose Weight?

- The mechanisms behind carb cycling suggest that it can be beneficial for weight loss.

- In theory, carb cycling may help you maintain physical performance while providing some of the same benefits as a low-carb diet.

- In contrast, many people may enjoy the flexibility of carb cycling. This could probably improve adherence and long-term success for some people.

- **Carb Cycling for Muscle Growth and Sports Performance**

- Many people believe that carb cycling can be beneficial for muscle gain and physical performance. The regular high-carb periods and targeted carb intake may help improve performance. Carbs around the workout may also aid with recovery, nutrient delivery and glycogen replenishment.

Introduction

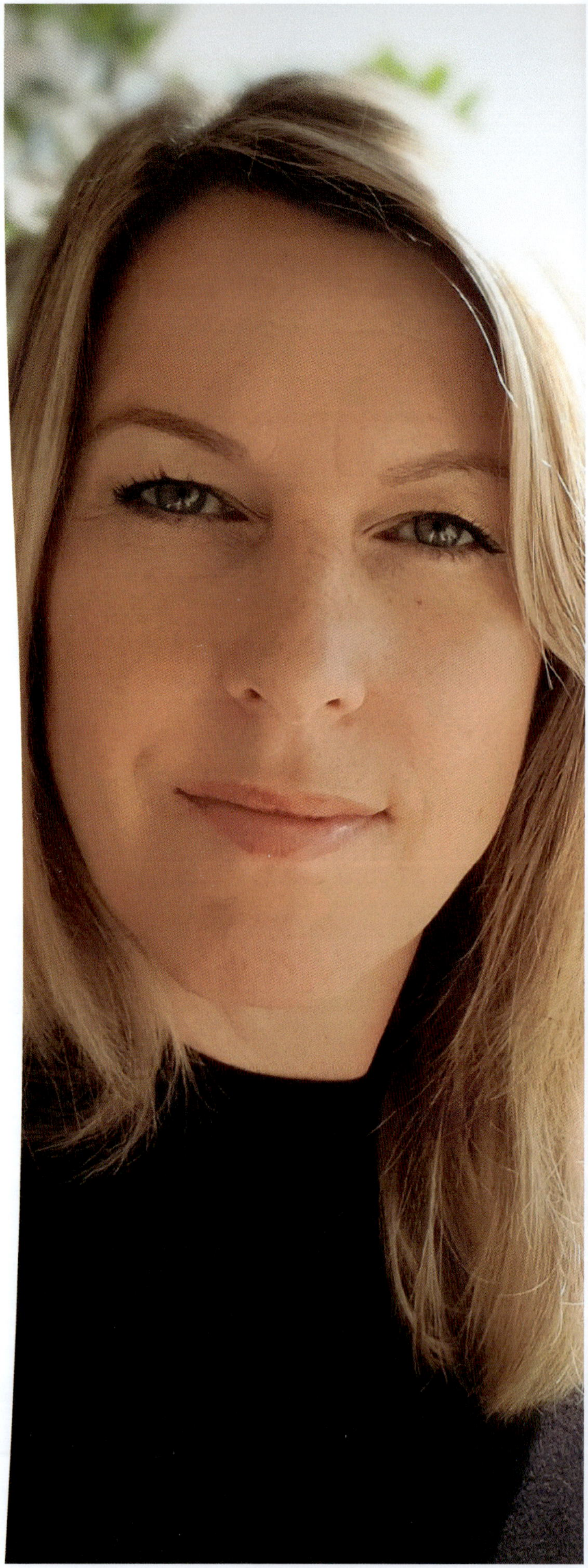

MY name is Kate, I am 42 years old and live in Malaga with my son, Luke, and husband Wayne. I started my own journey with carb cycling after seeing a few things on Facebook which pricked my ears up - a way I could eat my beloved carbs and still lose weight? Show me how!

After a couple of days of research and figuring out the formula to calculate my macros, I spent time pre-planning my meals for the week. It seemed pretty simple. And it was! I found I wasn't hungry or craving foods which I would usually miss out on a diet. I actually struggled to eat all the food at first, but my body soon adjusted to that! And the weight came off, pretty quickly. 4lb in the first week and maybe 2-3 a week after that.

I joined a few weight loss groups on FB and saw how many people were losing $$$ on impersonal weight loss programs. I started sharing my pictures and progress and people started to reach out to me to ask how I was doing it. So, I made my own group. I shared it on the group I was in and literally had 300 members in about a week. I couldn't believe it!
Members started messaging me, asking if I would make them a meal plan similar to what I was eating, so I did. I was offered 10$ so I figured it seemed fair. It took me about 4 hours - not the best hourly rate, but hey!

At the time of writing I have 12,500 members and growing daily. The page has over 18,000 followers and Instagram at 2,500 followers. All in less than 2 years.
I have met so many incredible people over this time, many of them inspire me to grow, to step back when I need to and most of all they inspire me and show me what is possible.
I hit my goal weight in two months of carb cycling, and 18 months later I am still the same weight. It is a way of life, not a diet, and I can't imagine eating any other way! So now it is time for me to share my most loved recipes from the last 2 years!

Thank you for purchasing or downloading the book and I hope it leads you on the journey you desire.
Good luck!

Kate

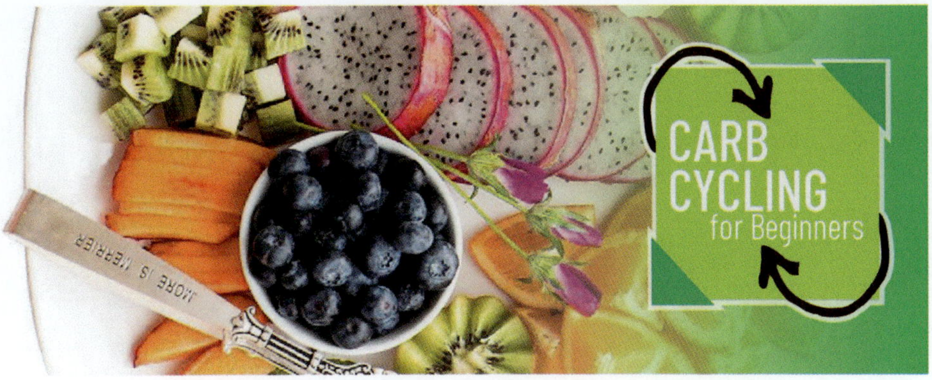

Party time!

THERE'S no shame in asking what alcohol you can drink on carb cycling, it is a way of life for many.

Dry wines, preferably white are very low carb, and so are clear spirits such as Gin and Vodka. Be sure to opt for slimline tonic on low carb day though as an average can contains up to 28g in carbs! Lagers and ciders are best avoided as the carbs are astronomical. A couple of cans and you will be close to your daily limit, even on moderate and high days!

One thing I always say to clients, is that its not always the actual drink you have which is the problem, It is the lower willpower this can bring. Once you have had a couple of wines, it is easy to believe that it is ok to start with the munchies and before you know it you will be raiding the cupboards!

If your tipple of choice is red wine, make sure it is dry and you can of course pair with cheese and nuts. But no crackers!

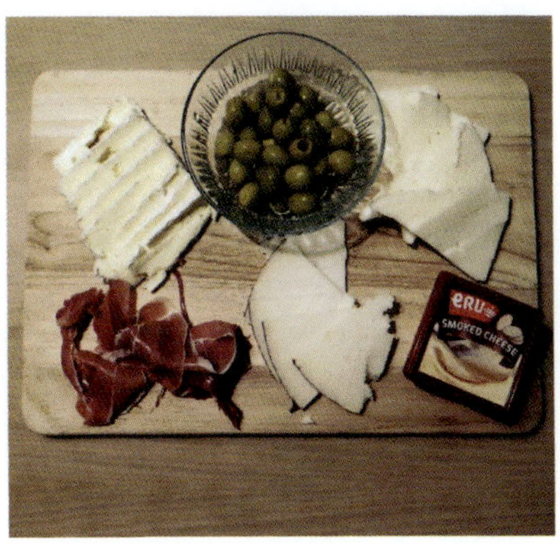

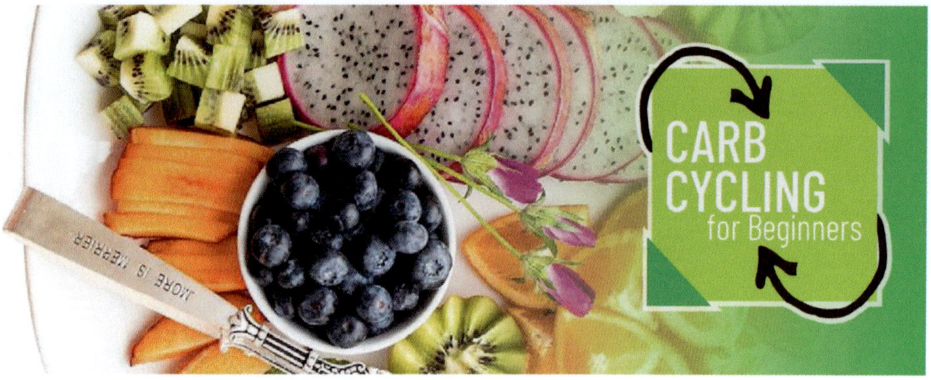

Top Tips

1. Never EVER skip high carb day. It is crucial to shock your metabolism.

2. Drink plenty of water and reduce as much salt in cooking as possible to shed any excess water weight.

3. Always get as close to your gram targets as possible! Calories are not the main goal here, the grams are.

4. Never do intense exercise on low carb days. Your body will demand carbs if you exercise and if you are on a low carb day it will store fat for energy.

5. Don't weigh every day. Your weight can fluctuate massively day to day especially in the first few weeks. Try to weigh weekly as a minimum frequency.

6. Take measurements. Non scale victories are important as carb cycling strips body fat and can show as inches instead of those pesky pounds.

Low Carb Days

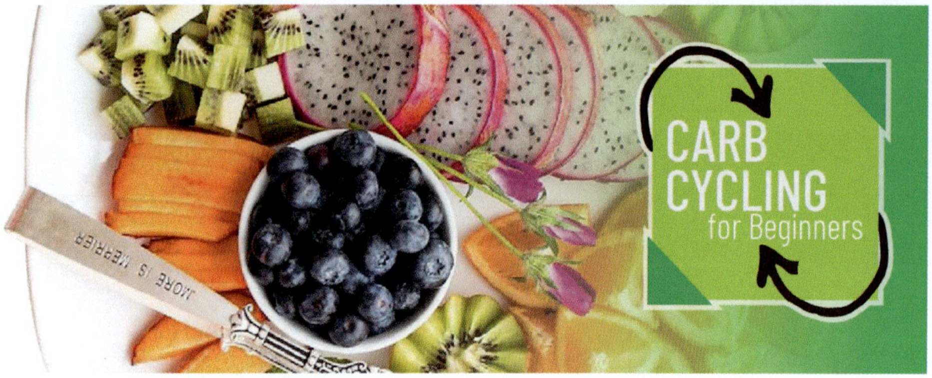

Low Carb Day

LOW carb day is the day everyone dreads at first, but grows to love more than the high carb days.

Why? Because most of us realise the things we love always include the fats! What good is toast without salty butter? Or pasta without cheese? Salad without a creamy dressing? The list goes on..

Low carb days are low in carbs (usually less than 50g) but more generous in fats. If you're a lover of cheese, meat fish and sauces then you will LOVE these days!

You will also find that these days are the days you are less hungry – you may even struggle to eat all the food. But get as close as you can, I promise it's ok!

No exercise on this day or you body will demand that you eat carbs and store the fat for energy instead.

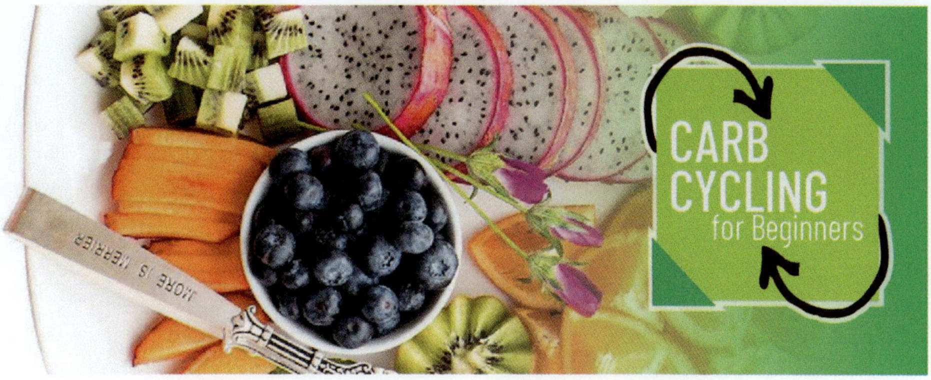

Low Carb Day

Essentials for your shopping list!

- Meat
- Fish
- Cheese (not processed)
- Full fat Greek yoghurt
- Berries
- Peanut butter
- Avocado
- Celery
- Red Pepper
- Butter
- Olive oil
- Nuts
- Eggs
- Heavy cream

Breakfast

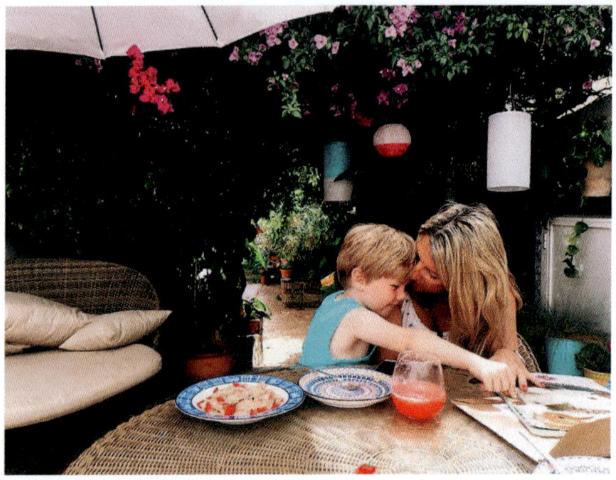

It is hard to create low carb day breakfasts without always resorting to eggs!

Of course they are easy, low carb and tasty, but it is also easy to tire of eggs quickly, so it is important to keep changing how you eat them!

I have also included some non egg recipes for those who don't eat eggs or have allergies.

Cheese and Veggie Fritatta

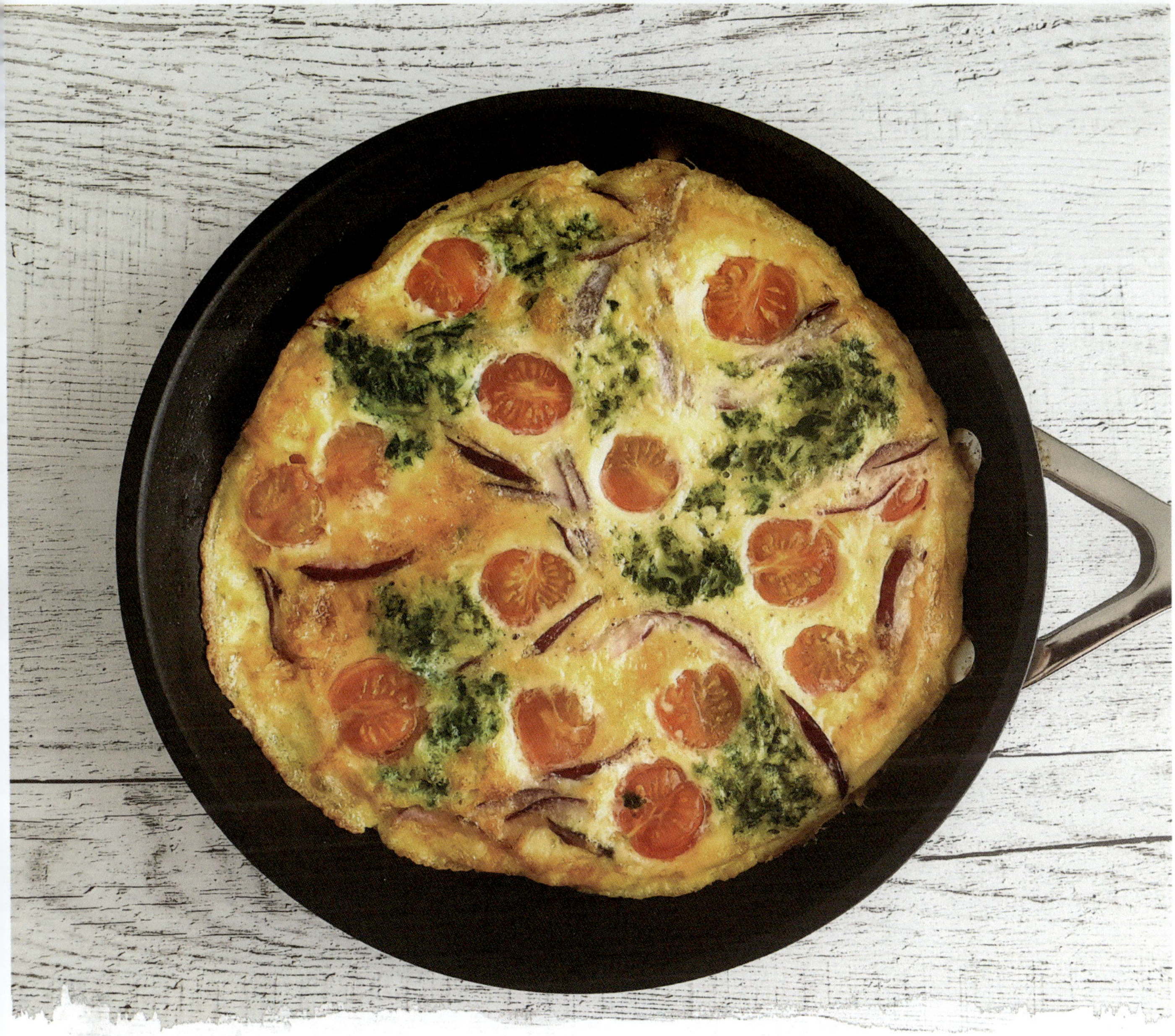

- 3 eggs
- 1 Tbsp Almond Milk
- Handful shredded cheese
- 6 Cherry tomatoes
- 1 Tbsp frozen spinach, thawed
- ¼ Cup Red Onion

Carbs 8g
Fat 31g
Protein 28g

Melt 1 tsp butter into a small frying pan.
Mix the eggs, milk and cheese and pour in.
Turn the heat to medium so as not to burn the bottom.
After a couple of minutes transfer the pan to a hot grill until brown and bubbling.

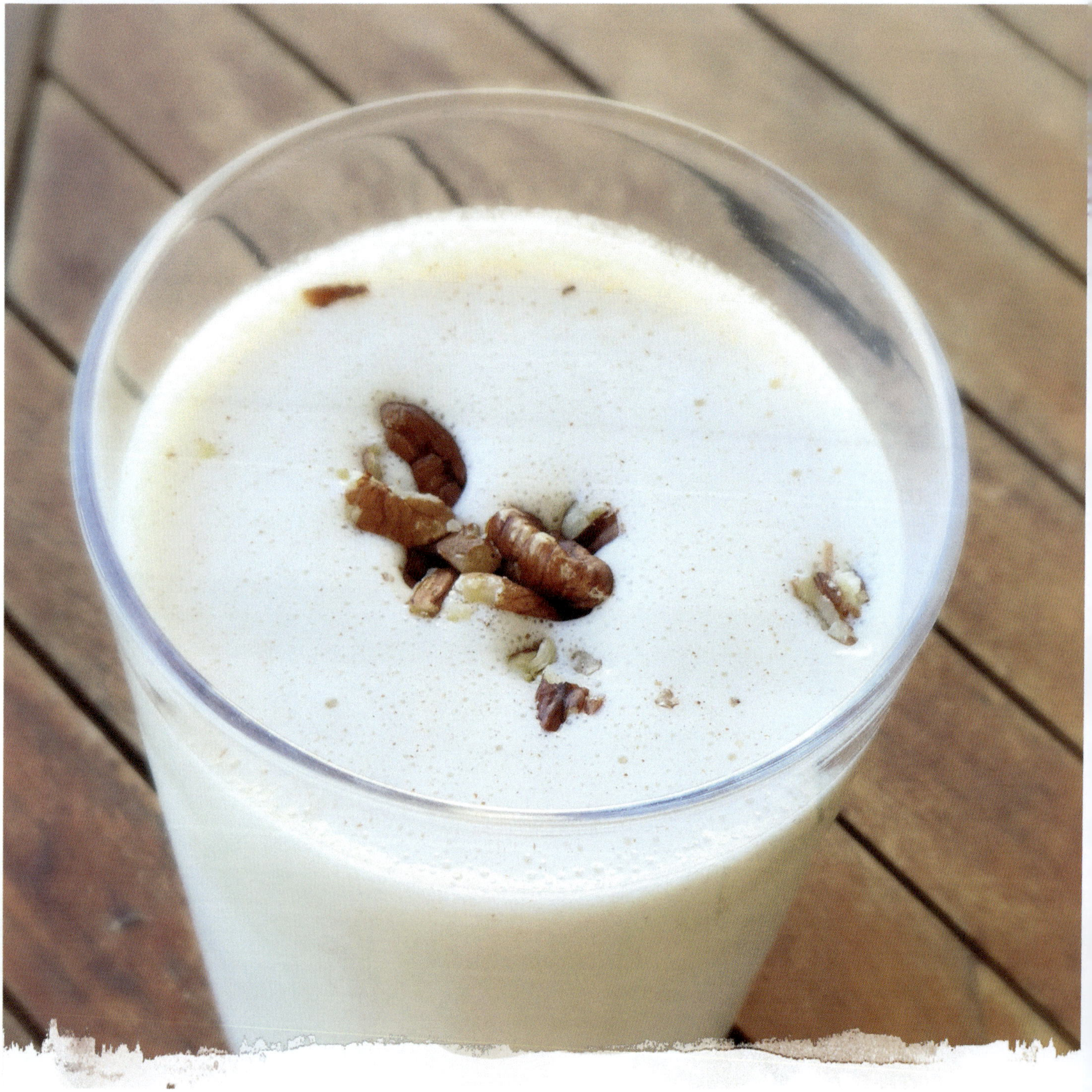

Breakfast Shake

- 1 Scoop vanilla protein
- 300ml Almond milk
- 1 Tbsp peanut butter
- 4 Pecans

Blend with ice in a high-speed blender!

Carbs 6g
Fat 26g
Protein 32g

Mediterranean Eggs

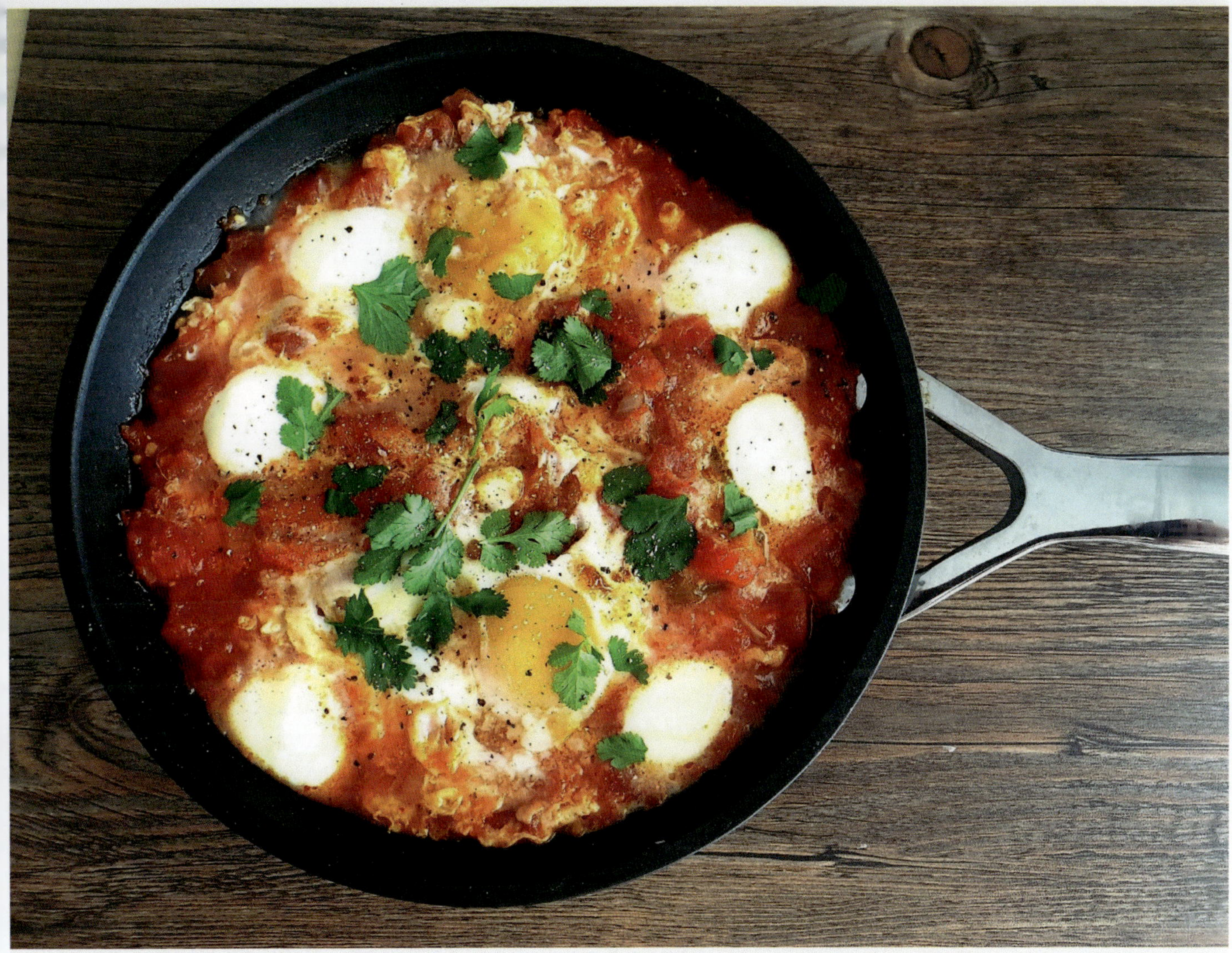

- 1 Can Tomatoes
- 2 eggs
- 6 Small Balls of Mozzarella
- 100g cooked red peppers, sliced
- 1 tsp butter
- Fresh Coriander/Basil

Warm the tomatoes and peppers with the butter, then add the mozzarella balls.

Make two small wells and crack in the eggs, cooking to your preference.

Garnish with fresh Coriander or Basil.

Carbs 11g

Fat 28g

Protein 23g

Maple Pecan Yoghurt

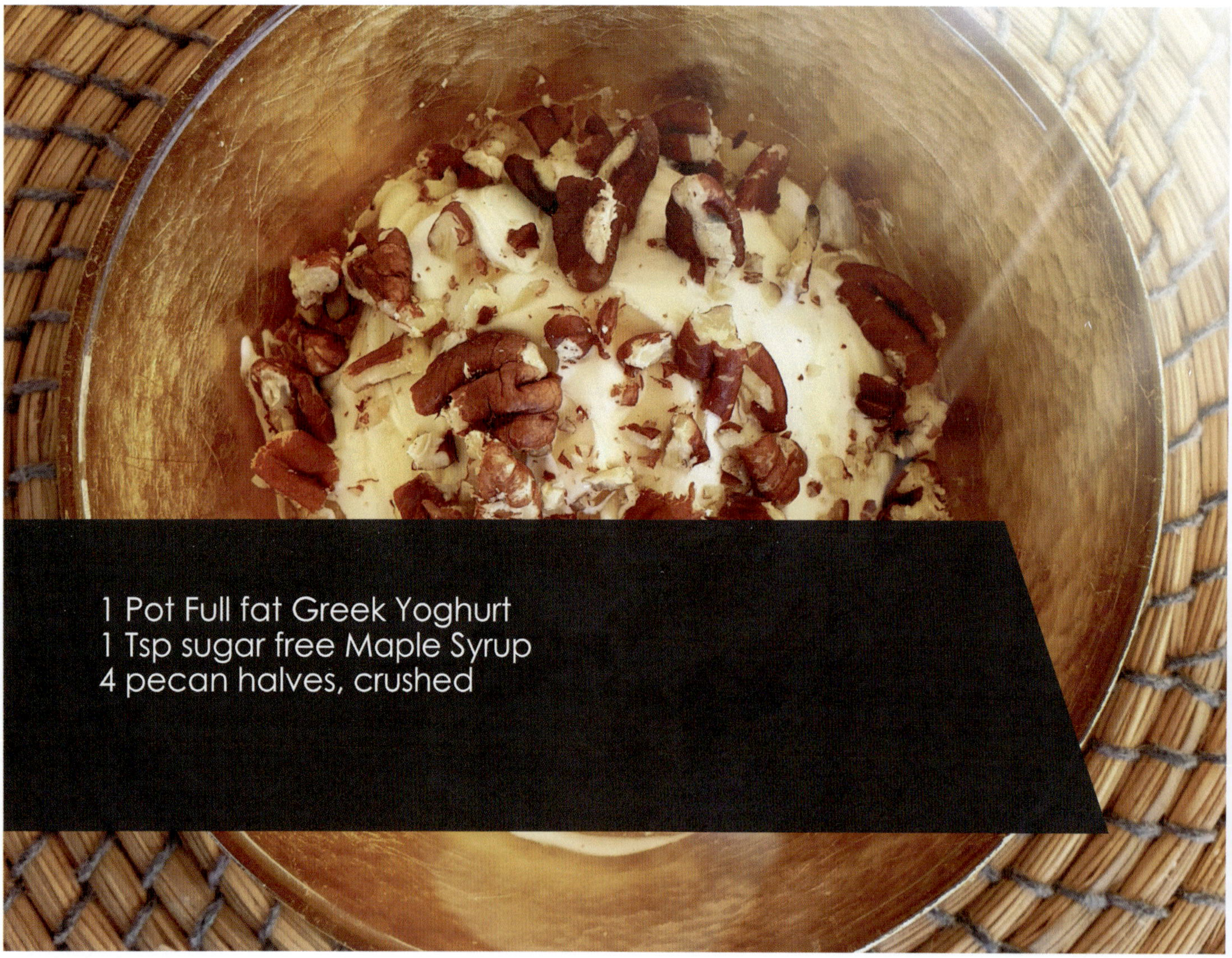

1 Pot Full fat Greek Yoghurt
1 Tsp sugar free Maple Syrup
4 pecan halves, crushed

Carbs 10g
Fat 30g
Protein 8g

Creamy Comforting Eggs

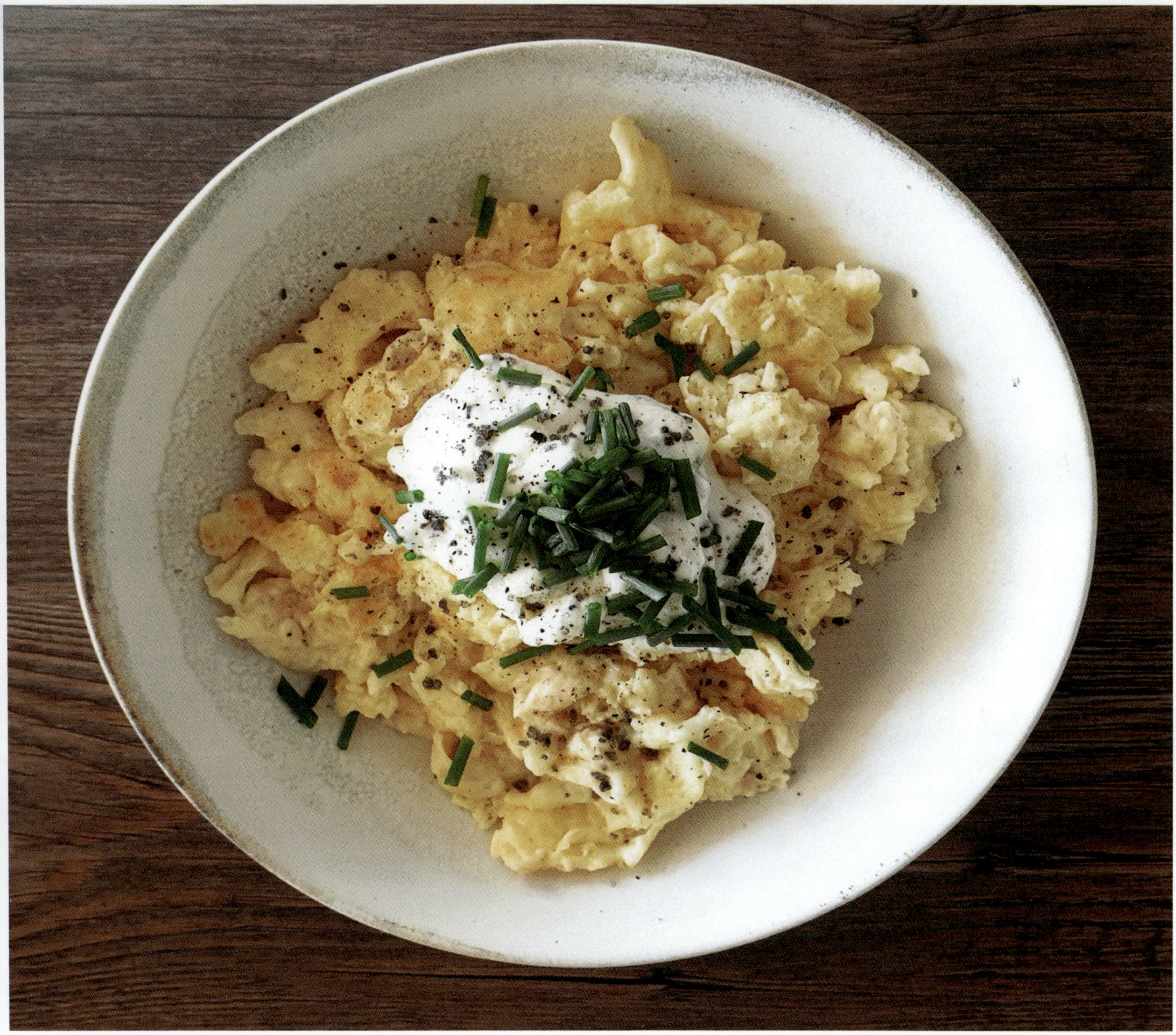

- 1 tsp butter
- ¼ cup Mozzarella
- 1 tbsp Fresh Sour Cream
- Chives, snipped

Carbs 4g
Fat 32g
Protein 25g

Melt butter in a small pan, being careful not to burn.
Add eggs and cheese, stirring constantly.
Serve with the sour cream and chives and eat right away!

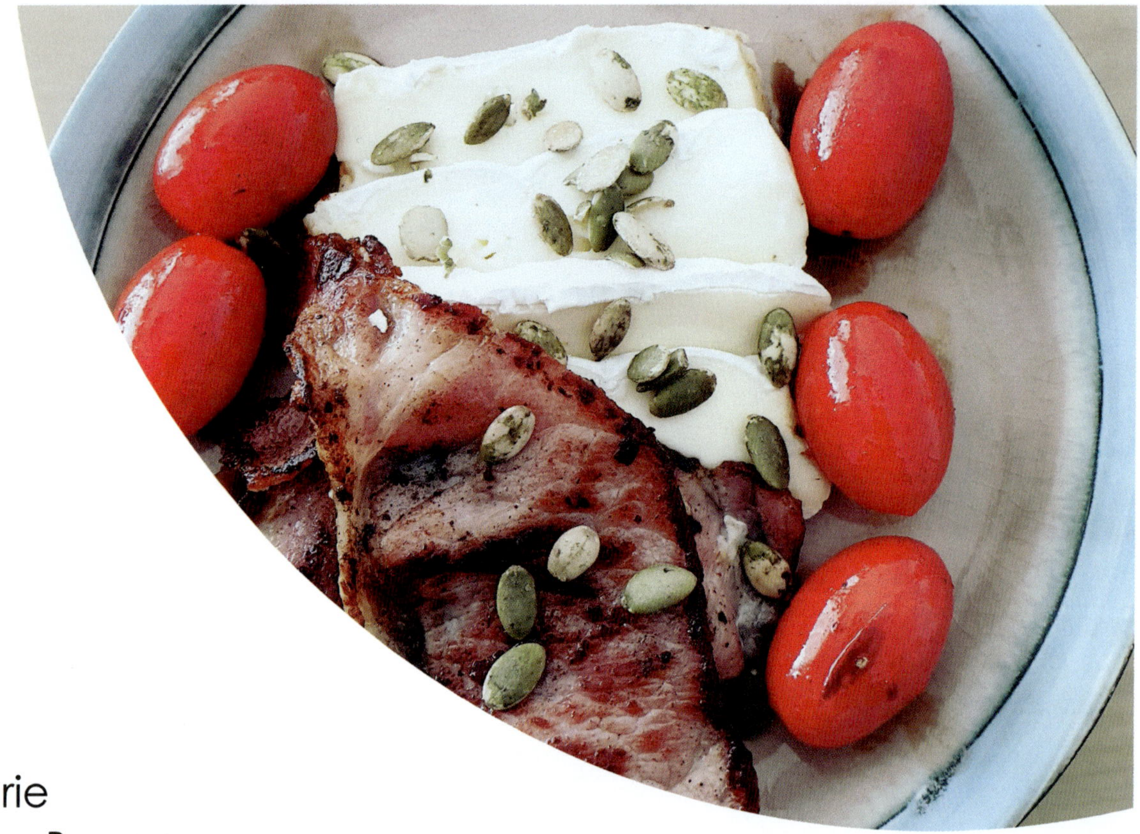

- 50g Brie
- 2 Slices Bacon
- 1 tbsp Pumpkin Seeds
- 5 Cherry Tomatoes
- Drizzle Balsamic Vinegar

Carbs 6g
Fat 30g
Protein 20g

Brie and Bacon Salad

Eggs 'n' Greens

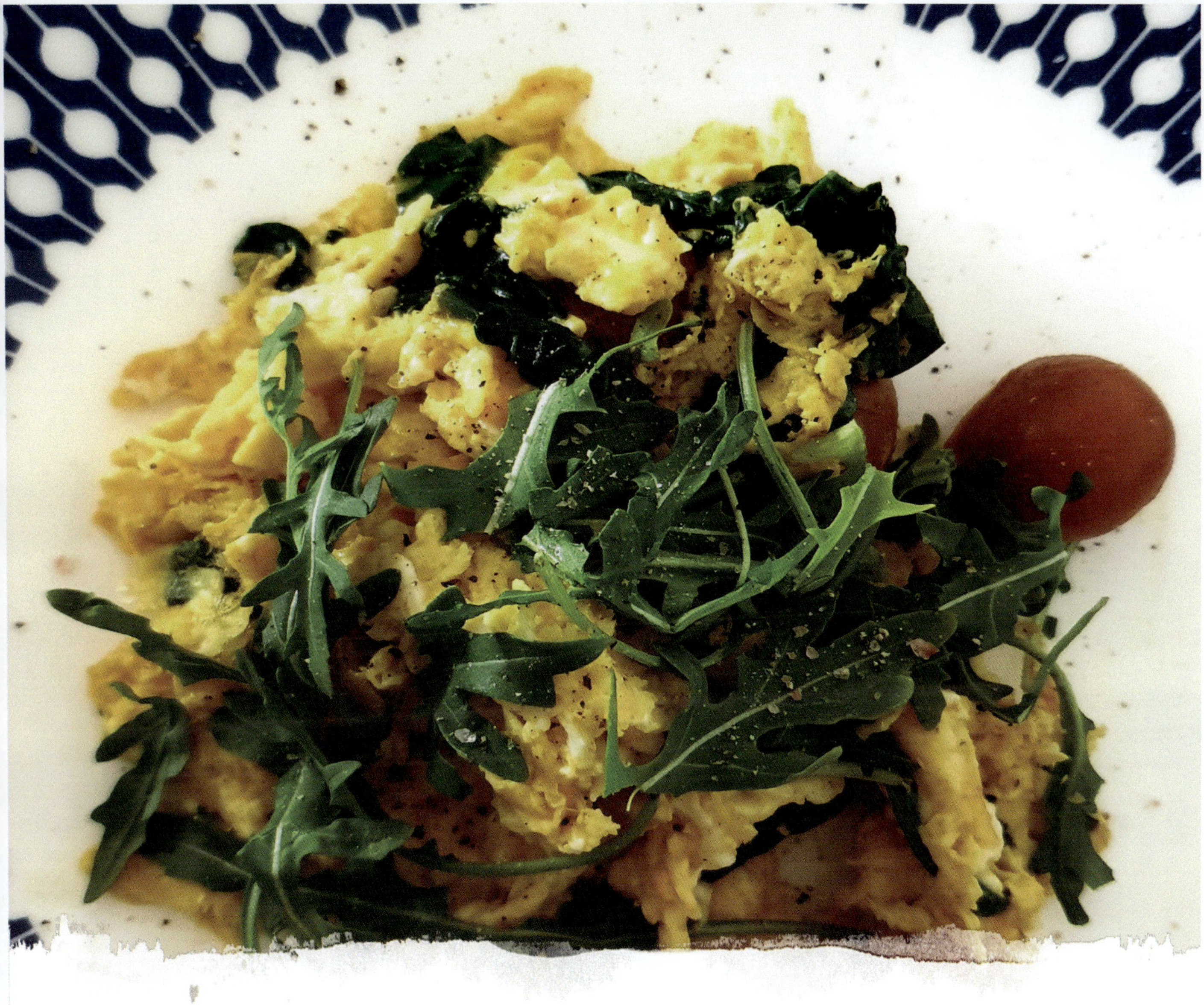

- 2 Eggs
- 4 cherry tomatoes
- 1 Cup baby spinach
- 1 Tbsp shredded cheddar
- 1 Tbsp butter

Carbs 7g
Fat 33g
Protein 25g

Gently melt the butter and add the eggs and cheddar. Separately, grill the cherry tomatoes until brown.
Wilt the spinach when the eggs are nearly cooked.
Garnish with arugula.
Season with sea salt and pepper.

Lunch

I prefer to have my biggest meal at lunchtime however I know this is not possible for everyone.

I have included a range of smaller and main meals for this section to also account for those who do intermittent fasting where this is the first meal of the day!

Roasted Vegetable Alfredo

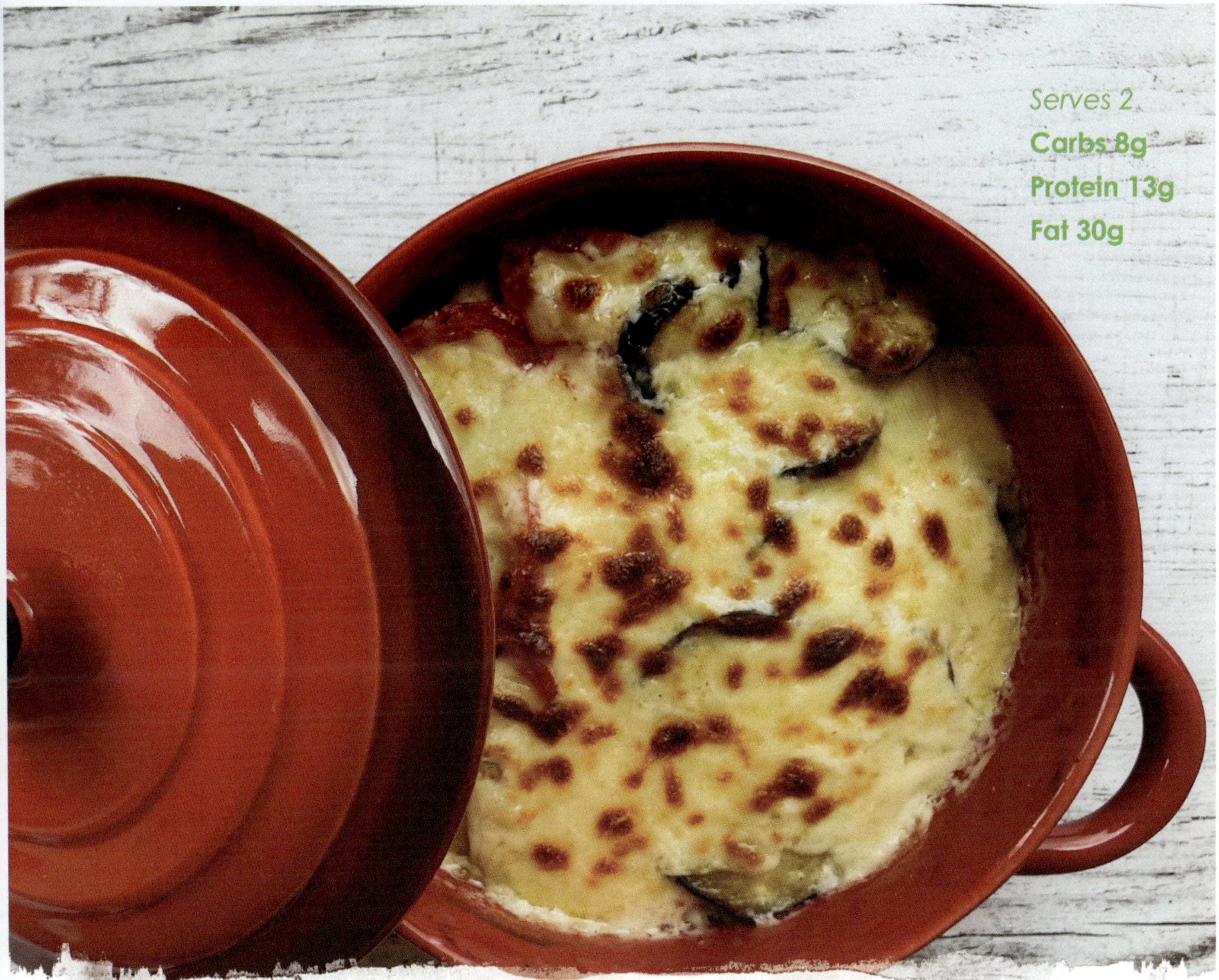

- Half a large eggplant sliced into thin discs
- One large pepper, sliced into rings
- 1 Tablespoon full fat cream cheese
- 100ml heavy Cream
- 1 Tsp Dijon mustard
- 1 tbsp butter
- 50g shredded sharp cheese
- 20g shredded mozzarella
- 1 clove garlic, crushed

Roast the veggies for approximately 15 mins until soft. Layer into an ovenproof dish.

Meanwhile, make the sauce, melting butter, then adding the garlic, sharp cheese, cream cheese, mustard and finally the cream.

Pour over the veggies and add the shredded mozzarella. Grill until bubbling.

Gambas Pil Pil

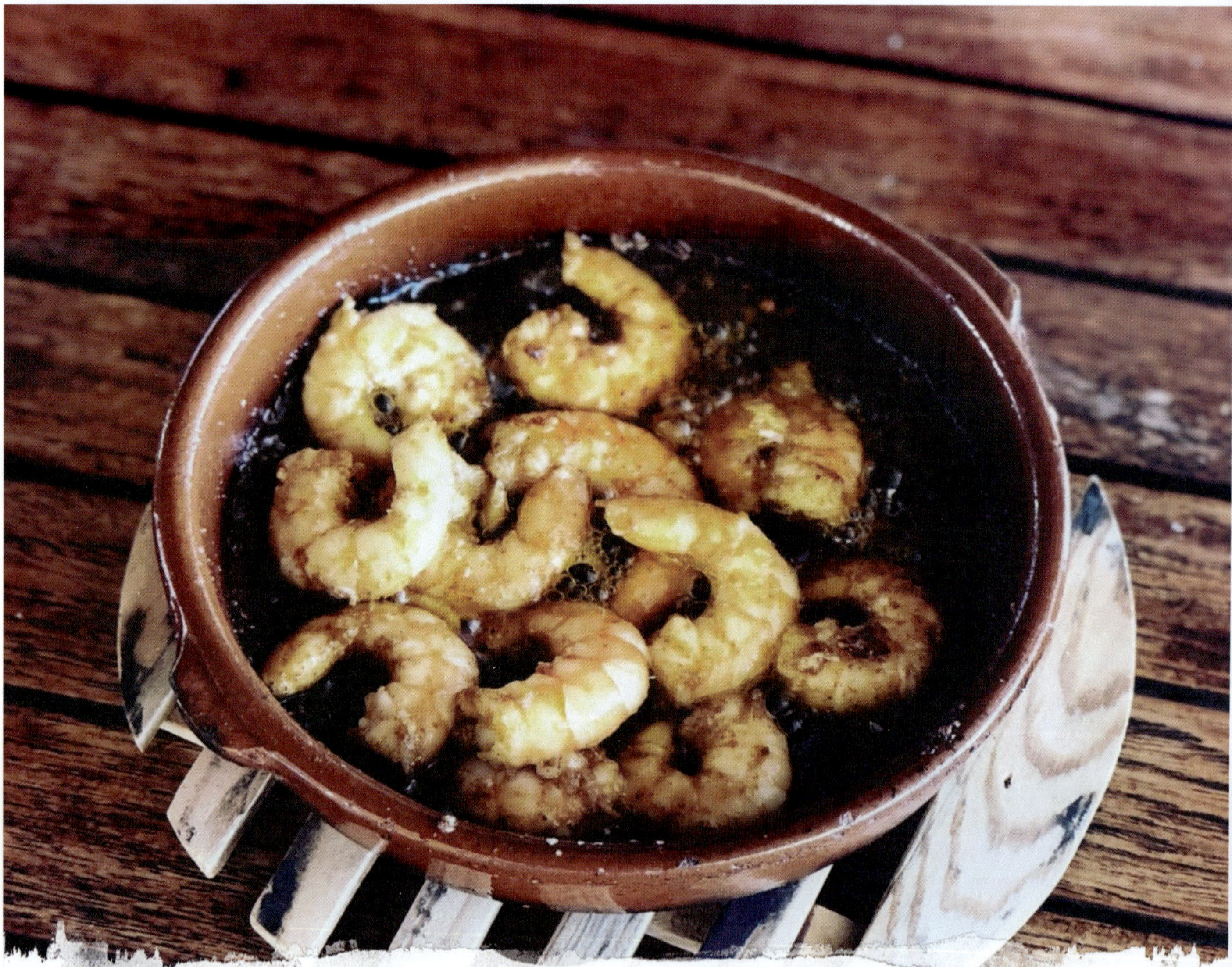

- 12 Medium fresh prawns, cleaned and de-veined
- 200ml Olive oil
- 2 Cloves garlic, chopped small
- Paprika/chili as your preference

Carbs 0.7g
Fat 28g
Protein 12g

In a terracotta dish, heat the oil with the garlic and any spices over a naked flame/hob.
Once the oil is sizzling, drop in the prawns carefully and leave to sizzle for 3 to 4 minutes until they are cooked through. Serve immediately. All of the oil will not be consumed, it will just coat the prawns.

Goats Cheese and Walnut Salad

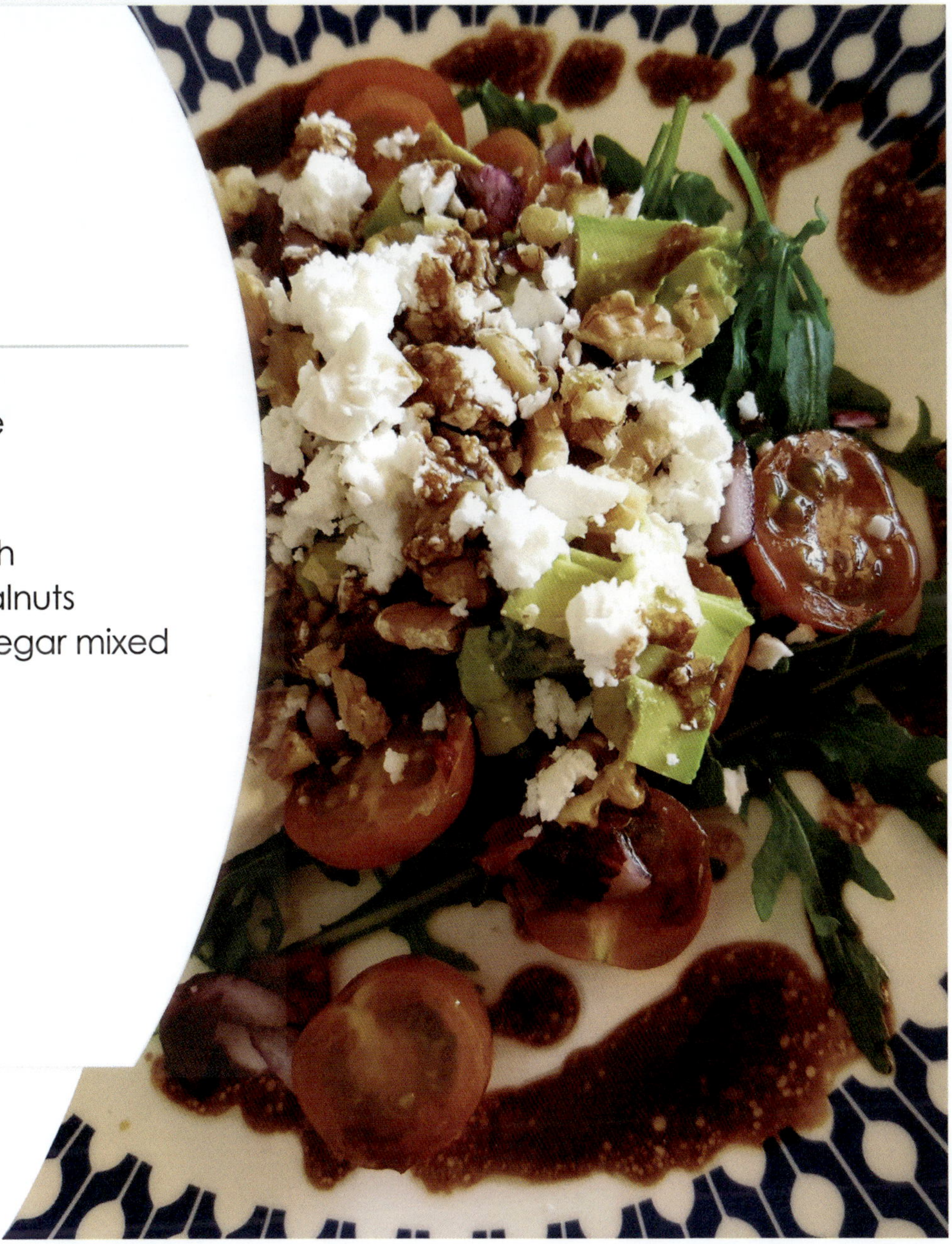

- 100g Goats Cheese
- ½ ripe Avocado
- 5 Cherry tomatoes
- 1 tbsp baby spinach
- 2 tbsp chopped walnuts
- 1 tbsp Balsamic vinegar mixed with 1 tsp olive oil

Carbs: 11g
Fat: 61g
Protein: 29g

Crustless Quiche

Serves 4

- 6 Eggs
- 1 Cup 1% milk
- 1 cup shredded cheese of your choice
- 1 cup additional ingredients (you choose and then add the relevant macros!

Preheat your oven to 350 degrees.

Whisk together the milk, egg, cheese and salt & pepper.

Stir in any additional ingredients.

Pour the egg mixture into a pie dish, and bake uncovered for about 45 minutes. Or until the centre is set, and not jiggly.

Carbs: 5g

Fat: 20g

Protein: 18g

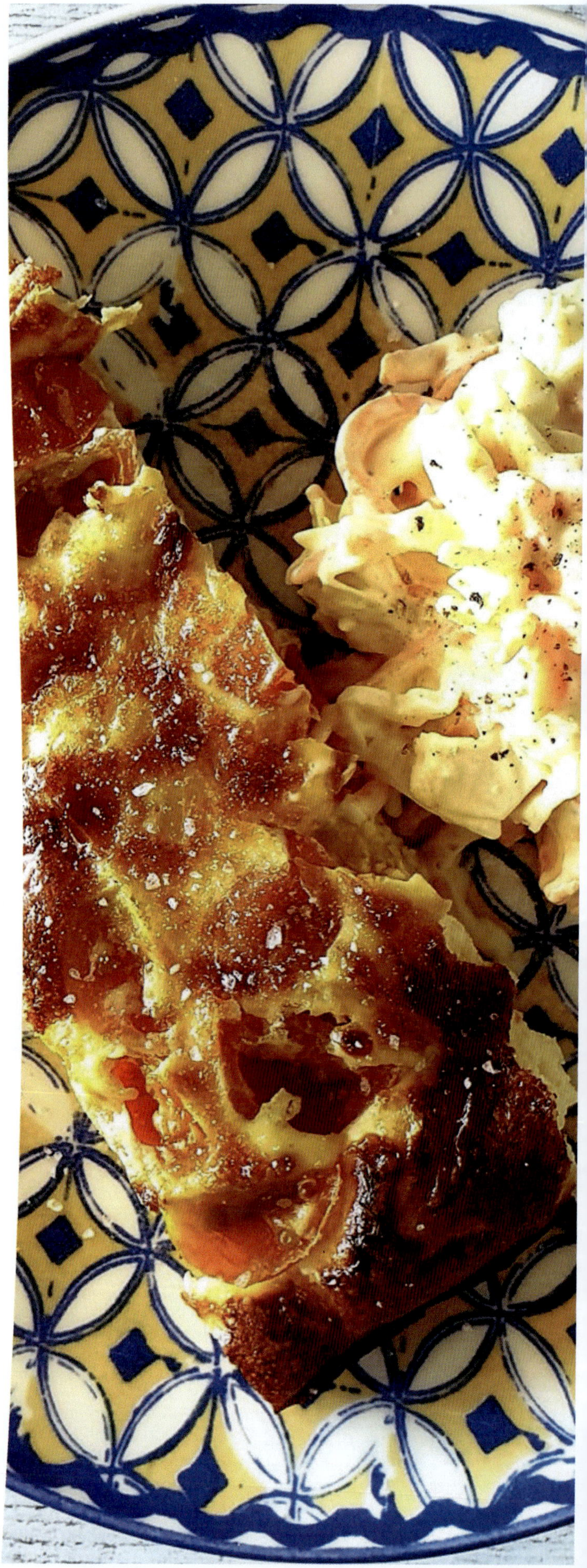

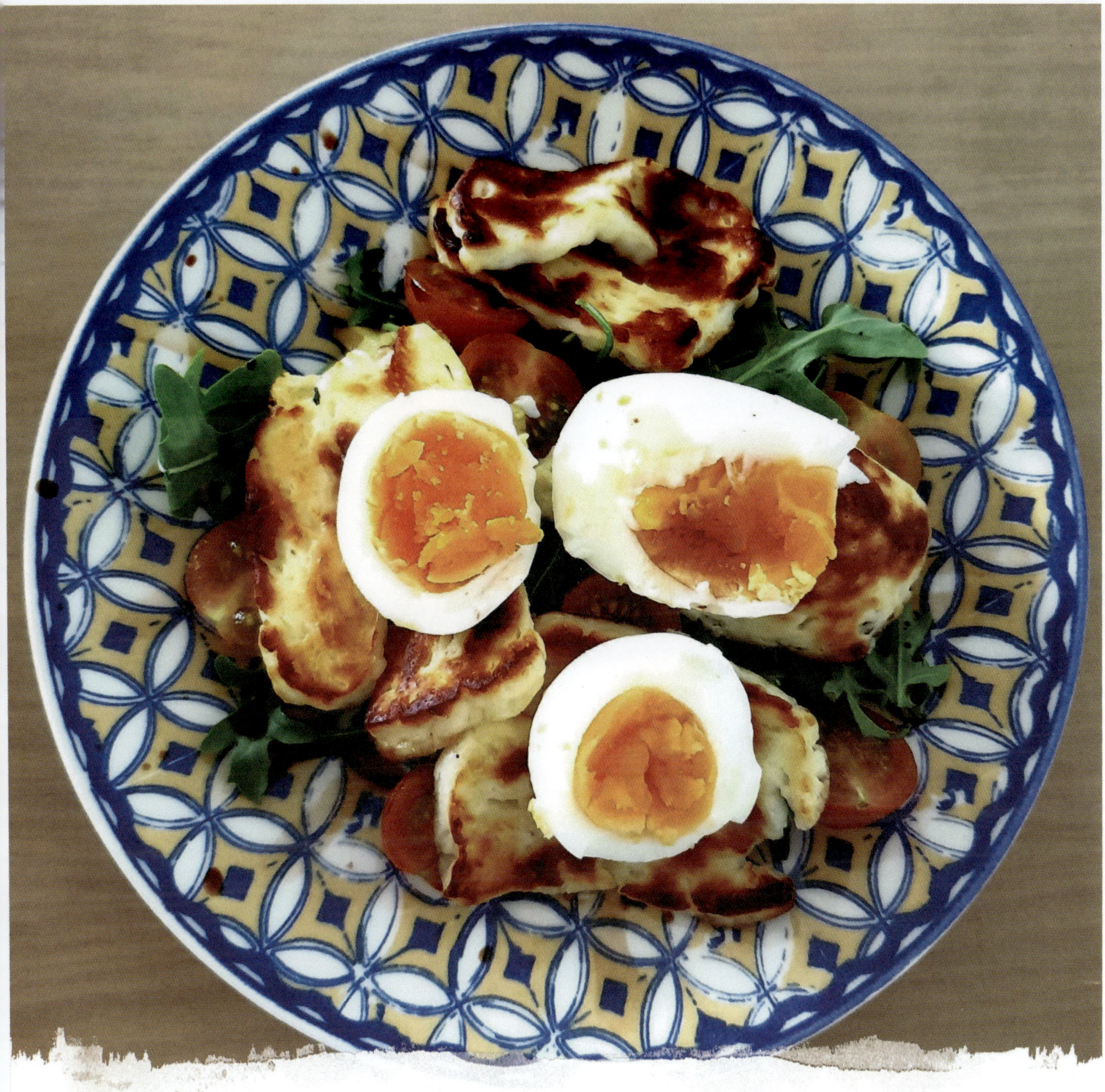

Egg and Halloumi Salad

- 100g Halloumi
- 2 boiled eggs, halved
- 4 cherry tomatoes
- 1 cup baby spinach or arugula

Carbs 6g
Fat 35g
Protein 35g

Simple Caprese Salad

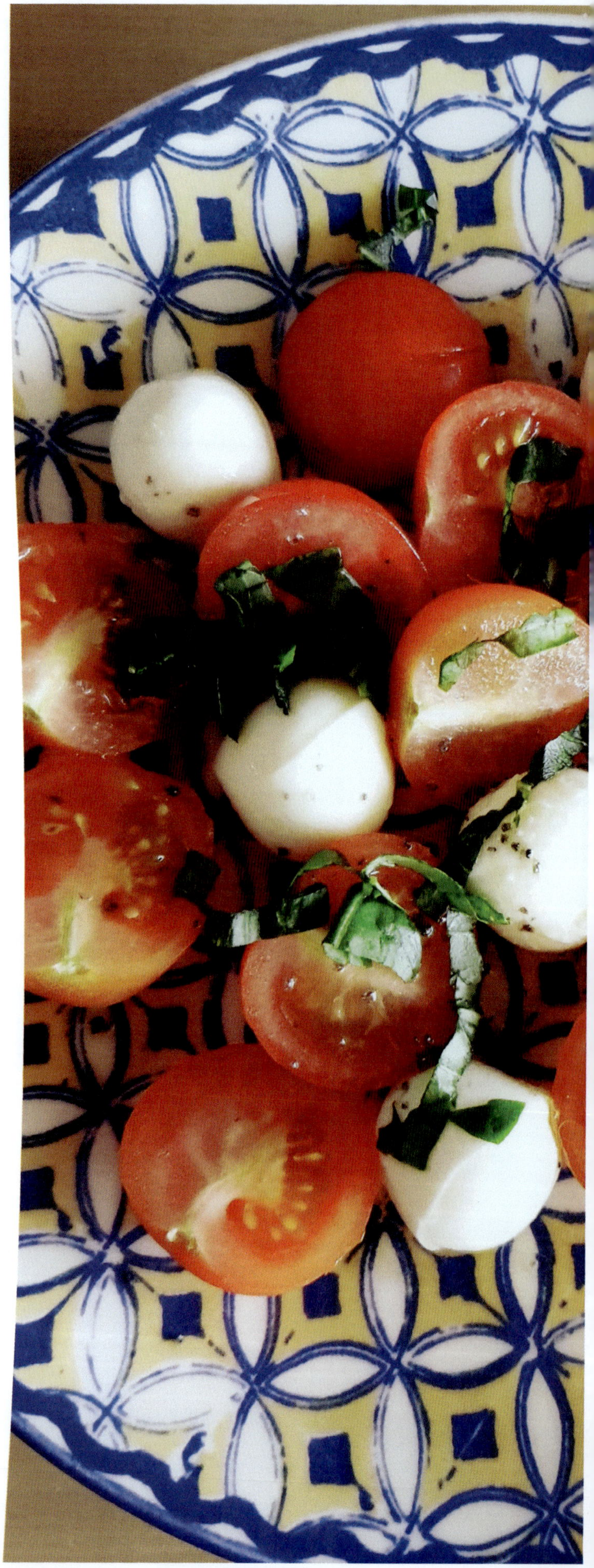

- 6 mini-balls of Mozzarella
- 6 Cherry Tomatoes
- Fresh basil, shredded
- 1 tbsp Olive Oil
- Himalayan salt

Carbs 4g
Fat 20g
Protein 8g

Zucchini Soup with Halloumi dippers

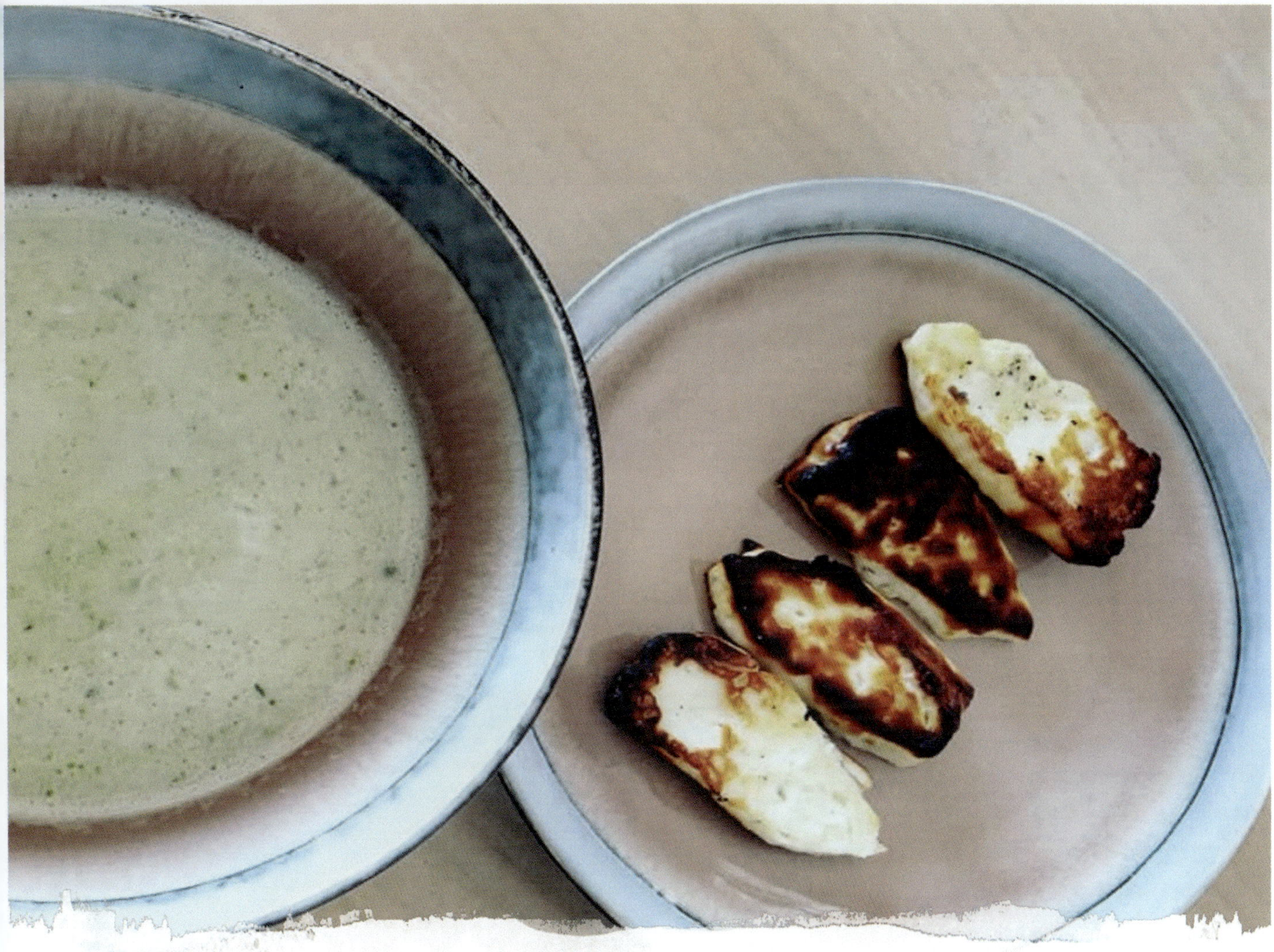

Serves 2

- 1 Whole Zucchini
- 1 Tbsp full Fat cream Cheese
- 200ml Water
- 1/2 Cup Halloumi cheese

Boil Zucchini until soft. Allow to cool, add the cheese and blend, reheating to serve.

Carbs 3.5g
Fat 4g
Protein 2g

Lightly Battered Cod Bites

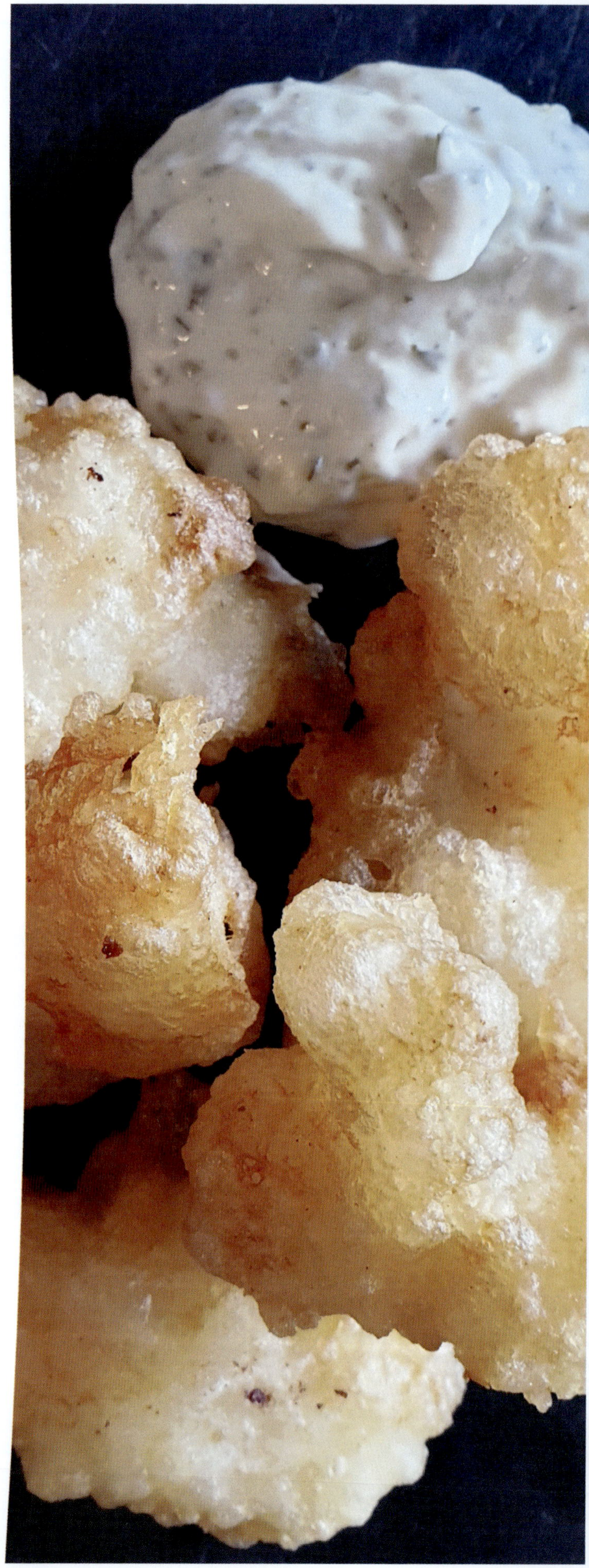

- 4 Small bite size cod or other white fish chunks
- 2 Tbsp flour
- 50ml Sparking sugar free water

Heat vegetable oil in a deep fat fryer to 180 degrees.

Mix the flour and water until a good batter consistency.

Dunk the fish into the batter and put directly into the oil (be careful!)

Cook for around 2 to 3 minutes until golden and bobbing around the top of the oil.

Serve with creamy tartar sauce or lemon wedges.

* **Not all of the batter will be used.**

Carbs 6g
Fat 15g
Protein 35g

Dinner

As this is the most likely meal to have with your family, all of the recipes listed are those which I have made for my son and husband, and hopefully you will agree they are suitable for those with a busy lifestyle and not a lot of time on their hands!

Try not to eat past 9pm in the evening to give your digestive system a chance to process your food, enabling a much better sleep!

Baked Cod with Zoodles

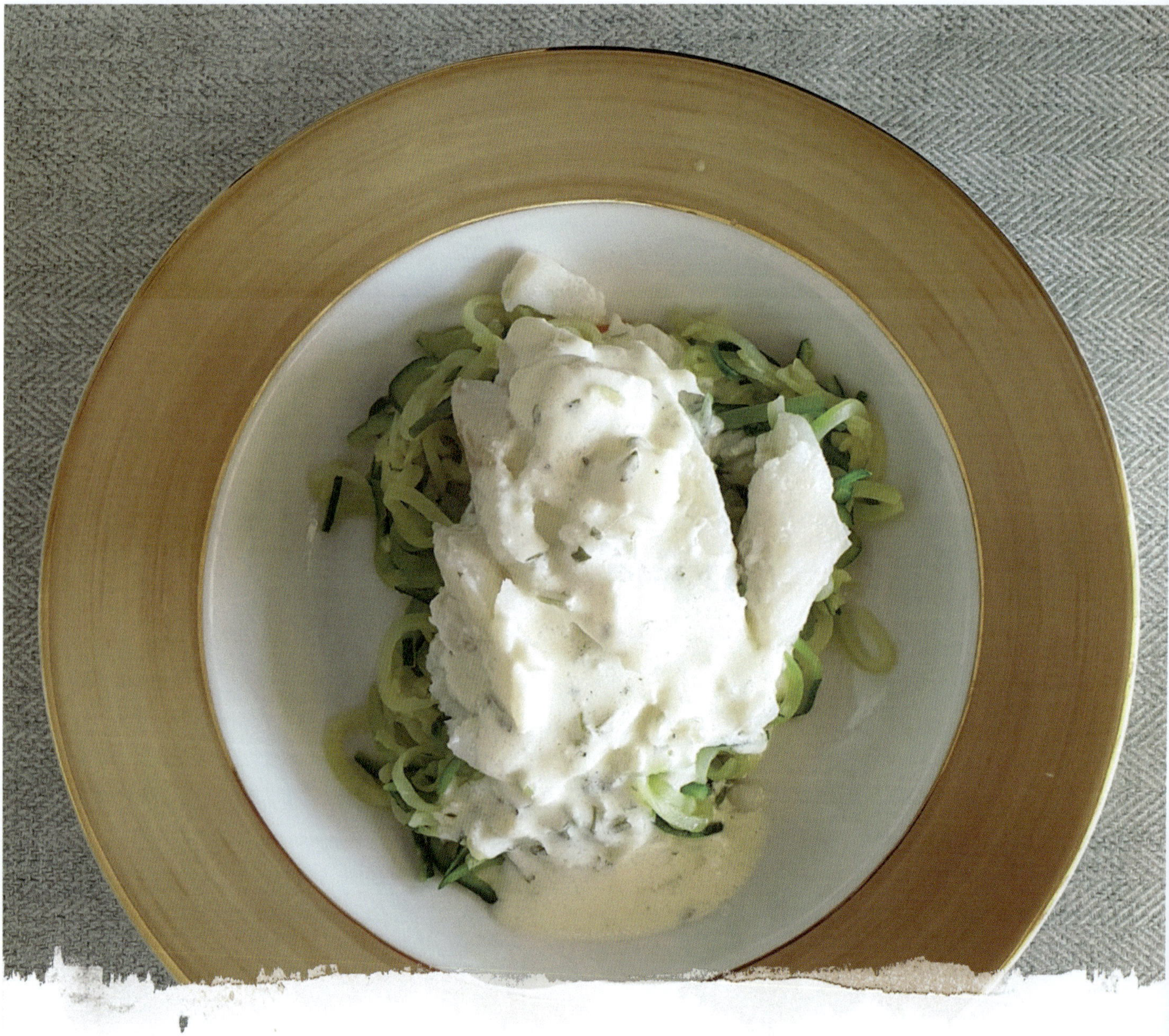

- 4oz Skinless cod fillet
- 200g Fresh zoodles
- 1Tbsp butter
- 1 Tbsp full fat cream cheese
- 1 Tbsp heavy cream

Bake the cod in the oven, wrapped loosely in foil, for 20 minutes.

Steam the zoodles until soft.

In a small pan, melt the butter, cream cheese and add the cream. Season to taste.

Carbs 7g
Fat 27g
Protein 38g

Celeriac Dauphinoise with Turkey and Buttery Cabbage

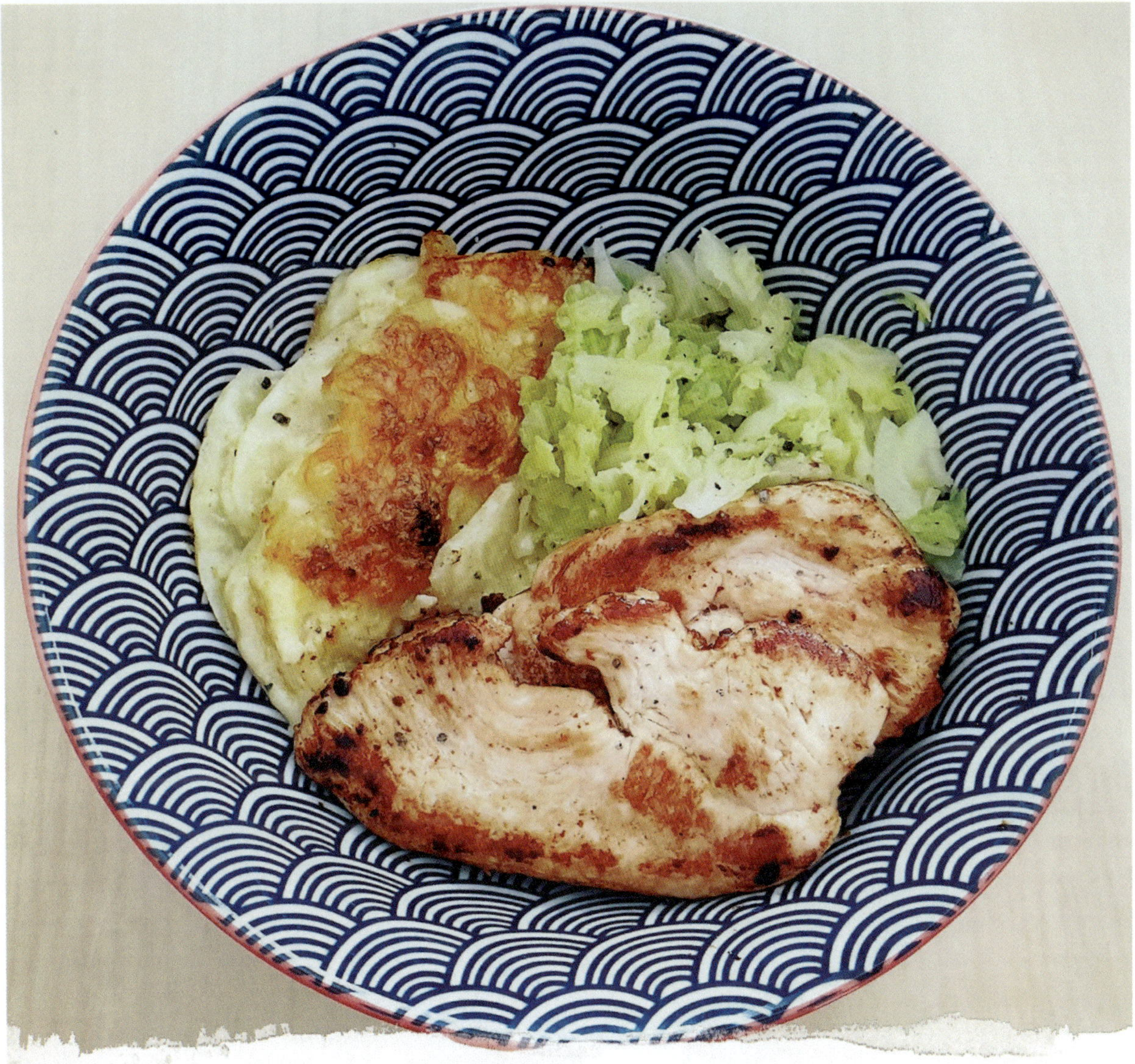

- 7oz Turkey breast
- 100g Green cabbage
- 100g Celeriac
- 75g Gruyere Cheese
- 50ml Heavy cream

Carbs 15g
Fat 41g
Protein 86g

Slice celeriac into thin slices. Place the slices in a large saucepan and add the garlic and cream. Place on the hob over a medium heat – The cream won't cover the celeriac completely but this is just to get the flavours introduced

Once simmering, cover and leave to steam for 5 minutes, then take off the heat and leave to cool slightly

Lift the celeriac out and arrange in a baking dish in layers, on top of each other. Pour the remaining liquid over the top and shake the dish so you have an even layer. Scatter over cheese and bake for 30 minutes or until the top begins to bubble and brown

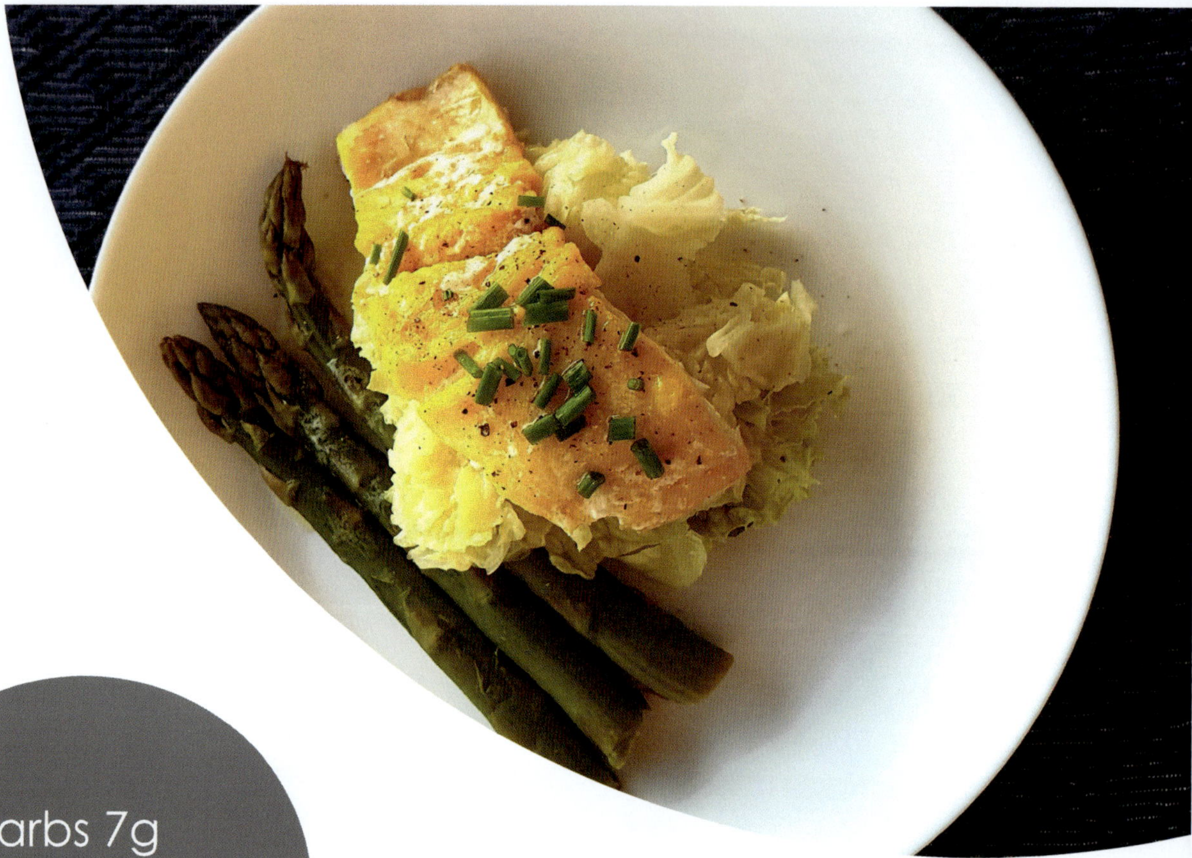

Carbs 7g
Fat 17g
Protein 19g

Smoked Haddock and Greens

Bake the Haddock for 20 minutes at 200 degrees, in foil.

3oz Smoked Haddock fillet, baked with lemon and butter
3 Spears of Steamed Asparagus
100g Cabbage, steamed
1 tsp Butter for the greens

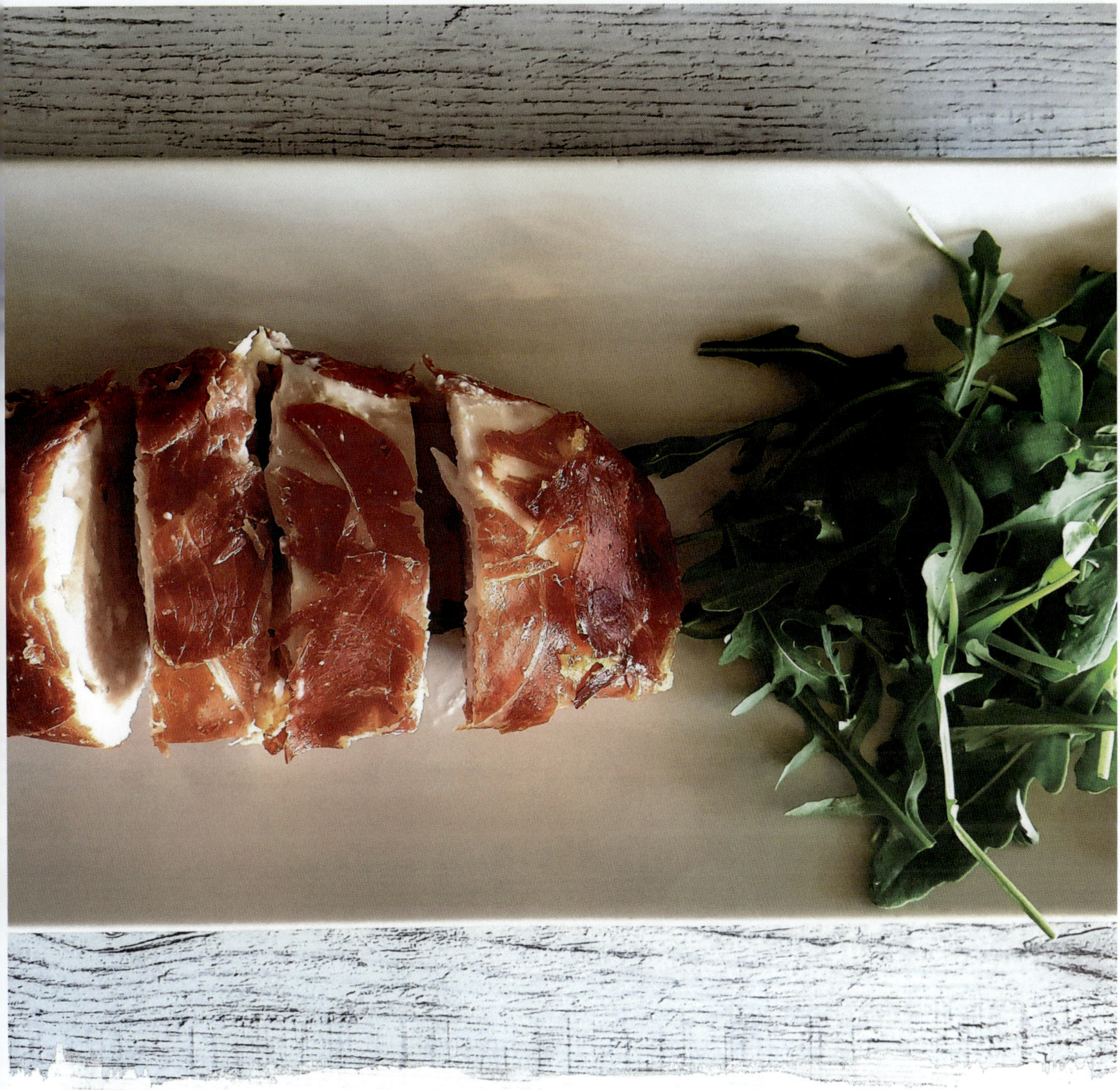

Bart's Philly Chicken

- 7oz Chicken breast
- 50g Serrano/ thin ham
- 1 Tbsp full fat cream cheese

Carbs 2g
Fat 17g
Protein 66g

Cut a pocket in the raw chicken breast and stuff with the cheese and garlic. Lay out the ham slices and place the breast on top, then wrapping around.
Bake the chicken for 15 minutes covered in foil, then uncover and continue for a further 15 minutes or until the chicken is cooked through.

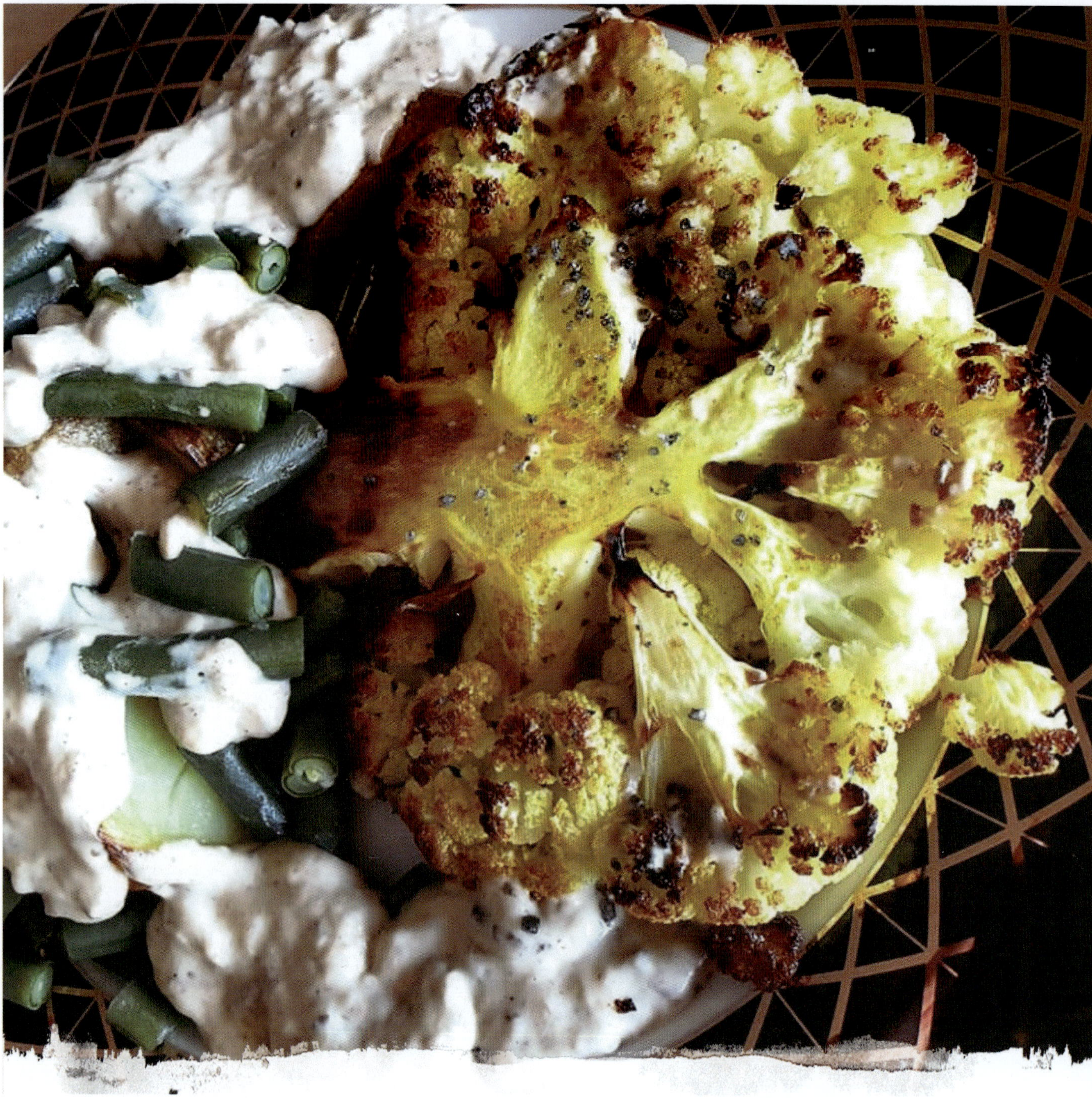

Cauliflower Steaks

- 1-inch wide slice of a full cauliflower
- 2 tbsp Olive Oil
- 1 Tbsp Garlic Paste
- 1 tsp Turmeric powder

Carbs 6g

Fat 20g

Protein 2g

- *Cook in a very hot oven for 15 minutes until golden!*
- *Serve with Roasted Veggies or your favorite meat or fish.*

Cheesy Chicken and Chorizo

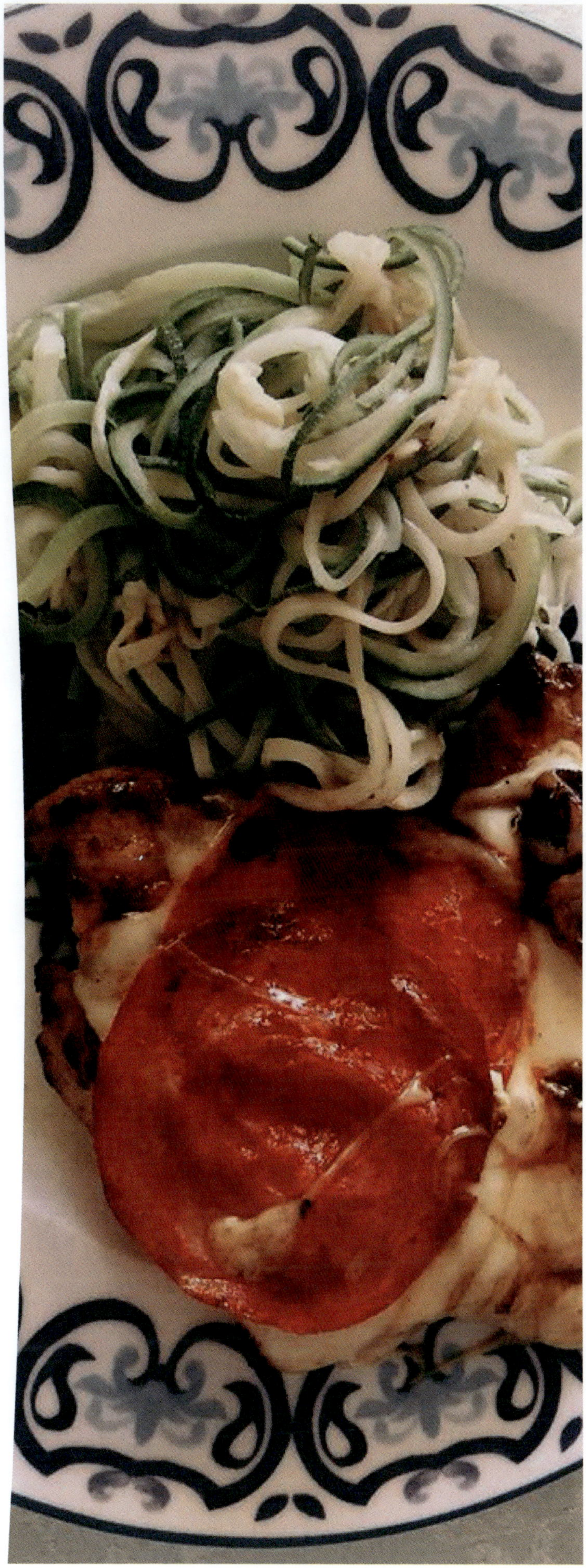

- 6oz Chicken Breast
- 2 Cheese slices
- 2 Slices thin chorizo
- 1 Cup Zucchini pasta

Pan fry the chicken on both sides until golden. Place cheese and chorizo on the chicken and put under the grill until brown and bubbling.

Steam the zucchini spaghetti to required texture.

Carbs 5.7g
Fat 15.4g
Protein 42.3g

Low Carb Lasagna

- 6oz Ground Beef
- 1 x Tinned chopped tomatoes
- 1 Whole red pepper
- ½ Medium Eggplant
- 2 Tbsp Grated cheese
- Fresh Basil or oregano
- Olive oil

Brown the meat in olive oil and add tomatoes and fresh herbs.

Meanwhile roast the peppers and Eggplant in olive oil, salt and pepper

Layer everything, add grated cheese and bake until bubbling!

Carbs 9.9g
Fat 18.1g
Protein 68.9g

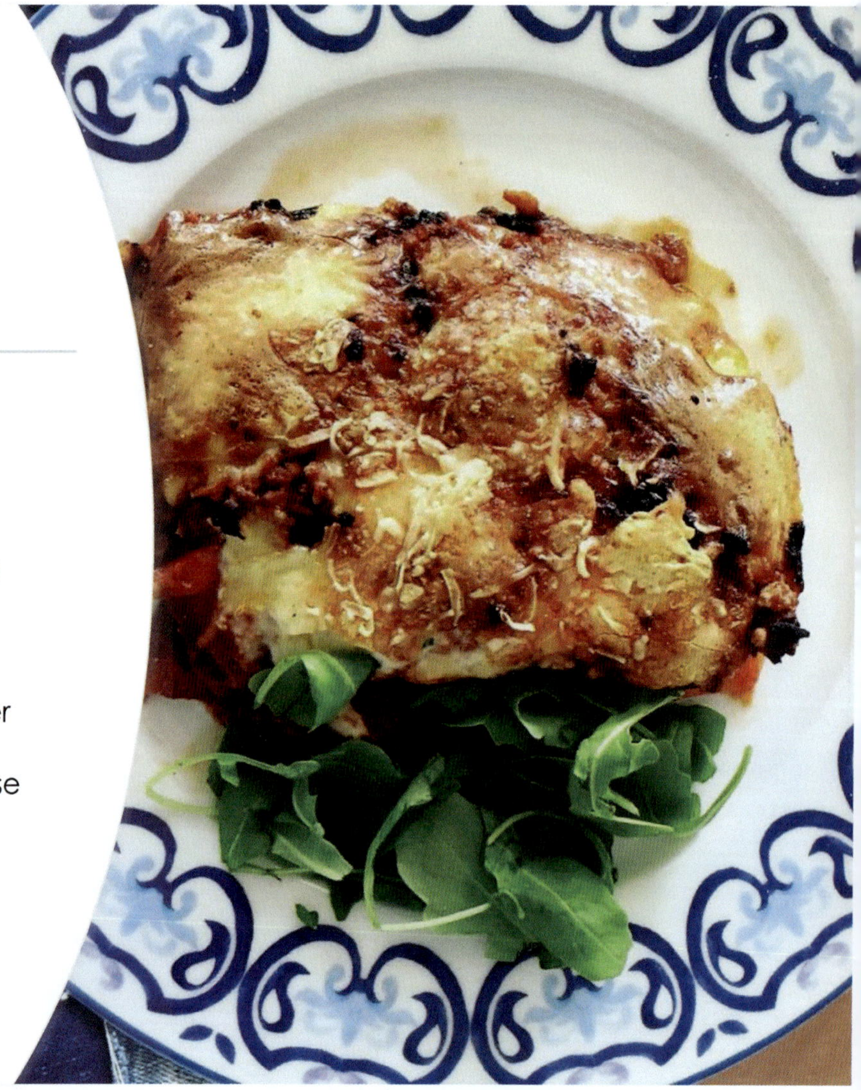

Pan fried veggies with Cauliflower Puree

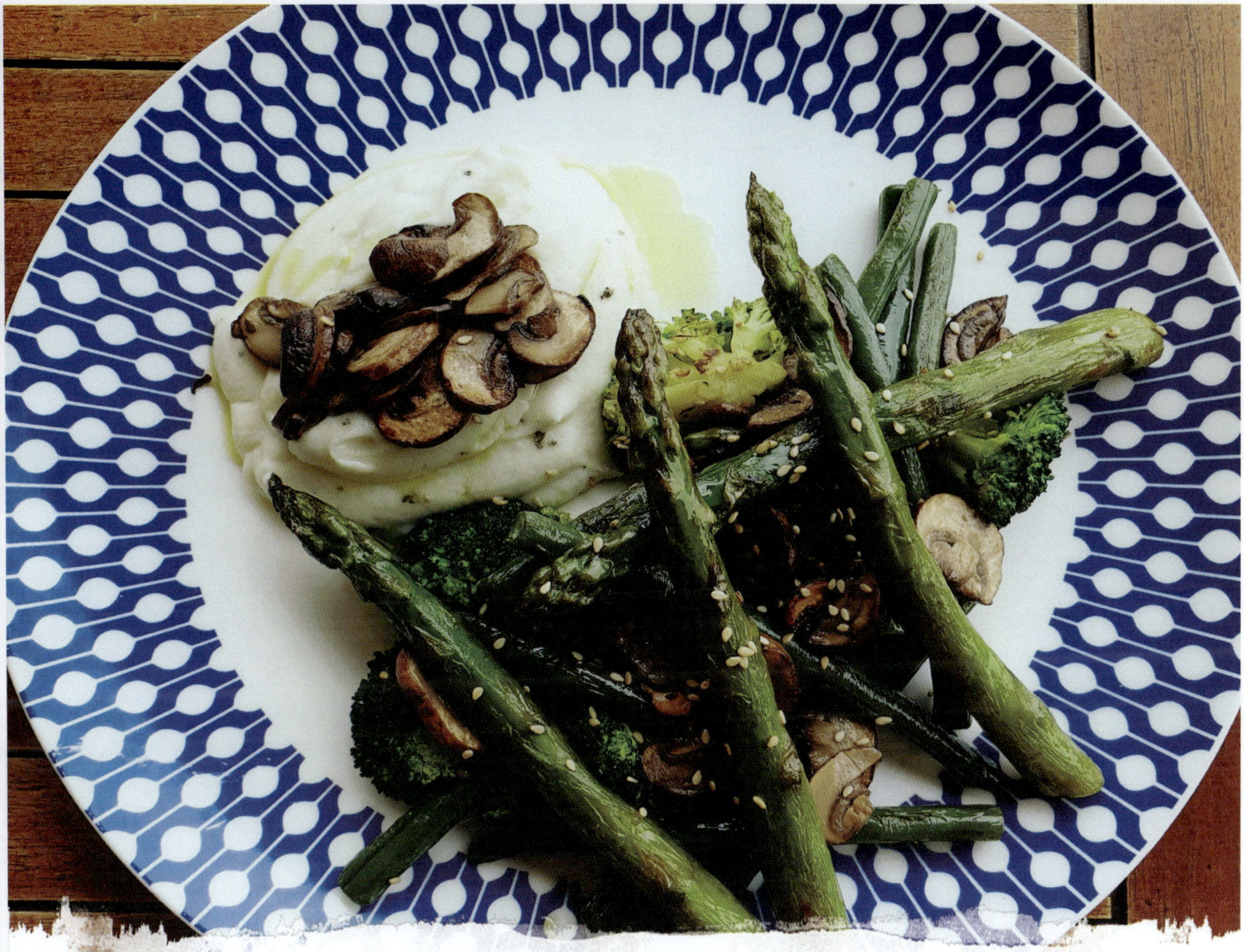

- ½ cup Portobello or Chestnut mushrooms
- 1 cup Broccoli
- ½ cup Green Beans
- 3 Spears of Asparagus
- 1 tsp Sesame Seeds

For the Mash:

- 1 cup cauliflower
- 1 Tbsp full fat Cream Cheese
- 1 tsp butter
- 15ml Double Cream
- ½ Clove Garlic

Steam all green veggies before pan frying

Fry the mushrooms separately.

Blend the mash mixture in a small blender.

Scatter the sesame seeds over the dish.

Carbs 19g
Fat 39g
Protein 18g

Creamy Chicken Spinach Curry

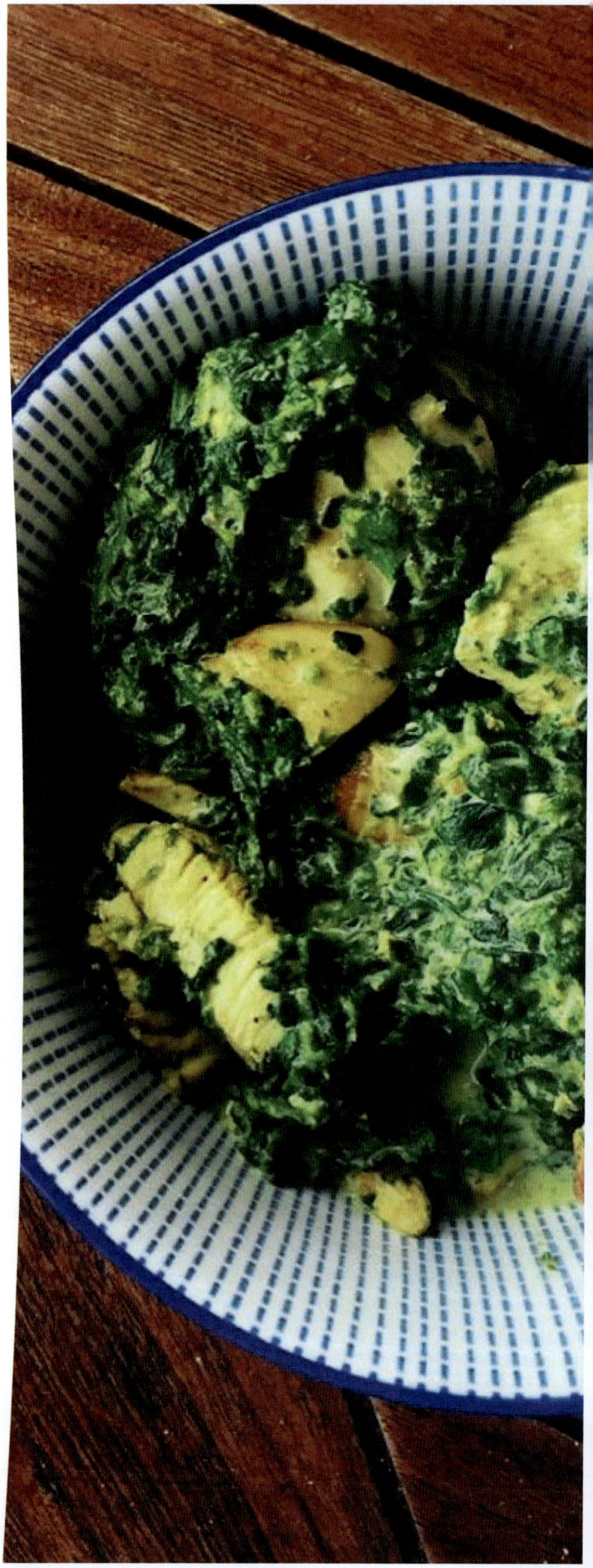

- 7oz Chicken breast, chopped
- 1 cup Frozen Spinach
- 3 tbsp Crème Fraiche
- Tsp Ginger
- Tsp Mild chili powder
- Tsp Turmeric
- Tsp Tandoori powder

Fry the chicken in olive oil until browned. Add the spices and 2 tablespoons of water. Add the defrosted spinach to the pan, including any liquid.

Turn the heat low and simmer for 5 minutes, then add the crème fraiche.

Carbs 5g

Fat 26.4g

Protein 69.6g

Pan Fried Turkey Supreme

- 6oz Chicken or turkey breast steaks
- ½ Cup Mushrooms
- 1 Clove Garlic
- 1 Tbsp Butter
- ½ cup Heavy Cream

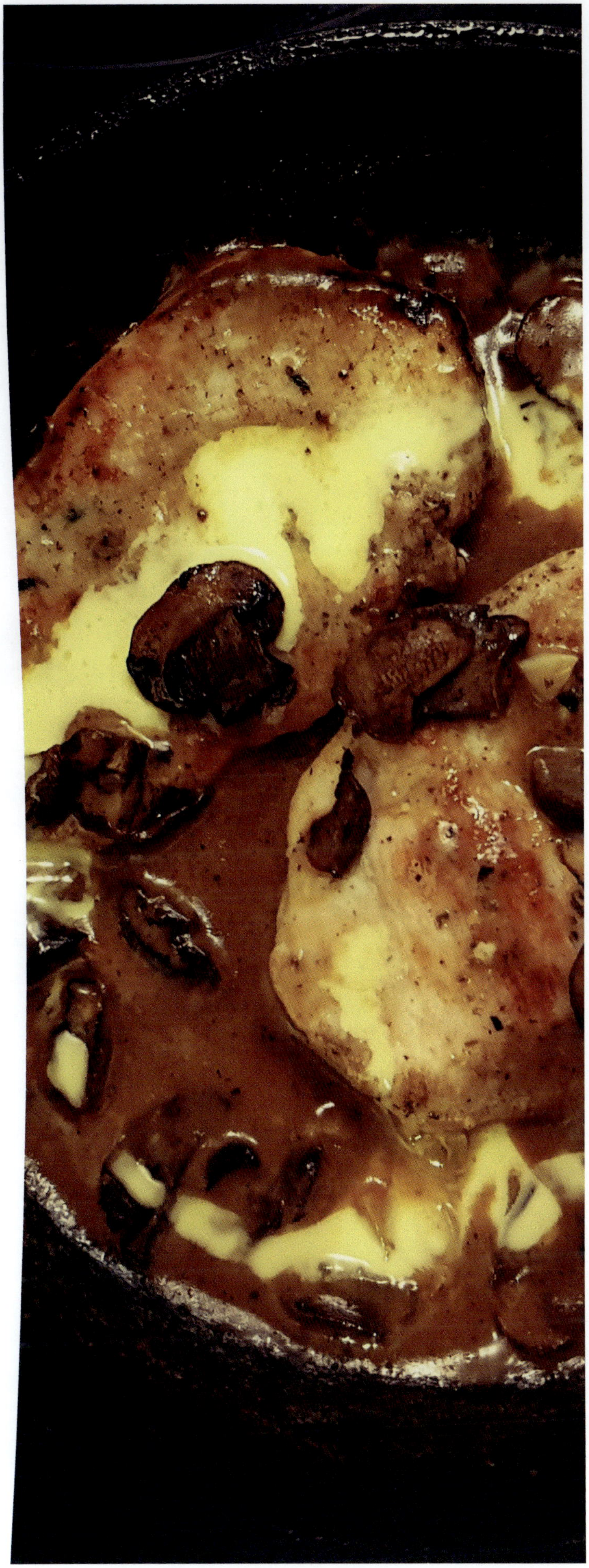

Fry the chicken, garlic and mushrooms until golden and the chicken is almost cooked through.

Turn the heat low and add the cream and simmer until the chicken is fully cooked.

Carbs 1g
Fat 20g
Protein 62g

Spicy Beef with mustard dip

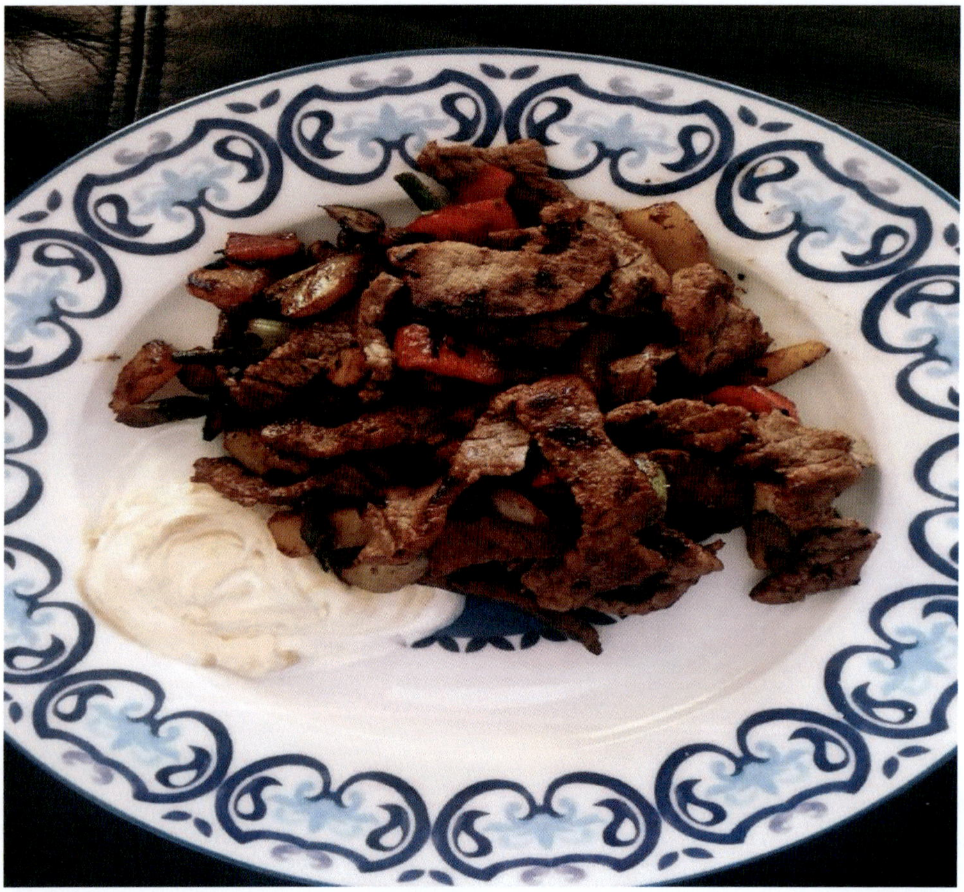

Serves 2

- 6oz Sliced fillet of Beef
- 1 cup Sliced red and yellow
- peppers
- 1 tsp mild chili powder
- 1 clove crushed garlic
- 2 tbsp Crème Fraiche
- 1 Tsp dijon mustard

Fry the steak and peppers with garlic and chili powder until browned and peppers are soft.

Mix the crème fraiche with the mustard until blended

Carbs 8.6g, Fat 9.8g, Protein 38.9g

Baked Cod with Steamed Greens

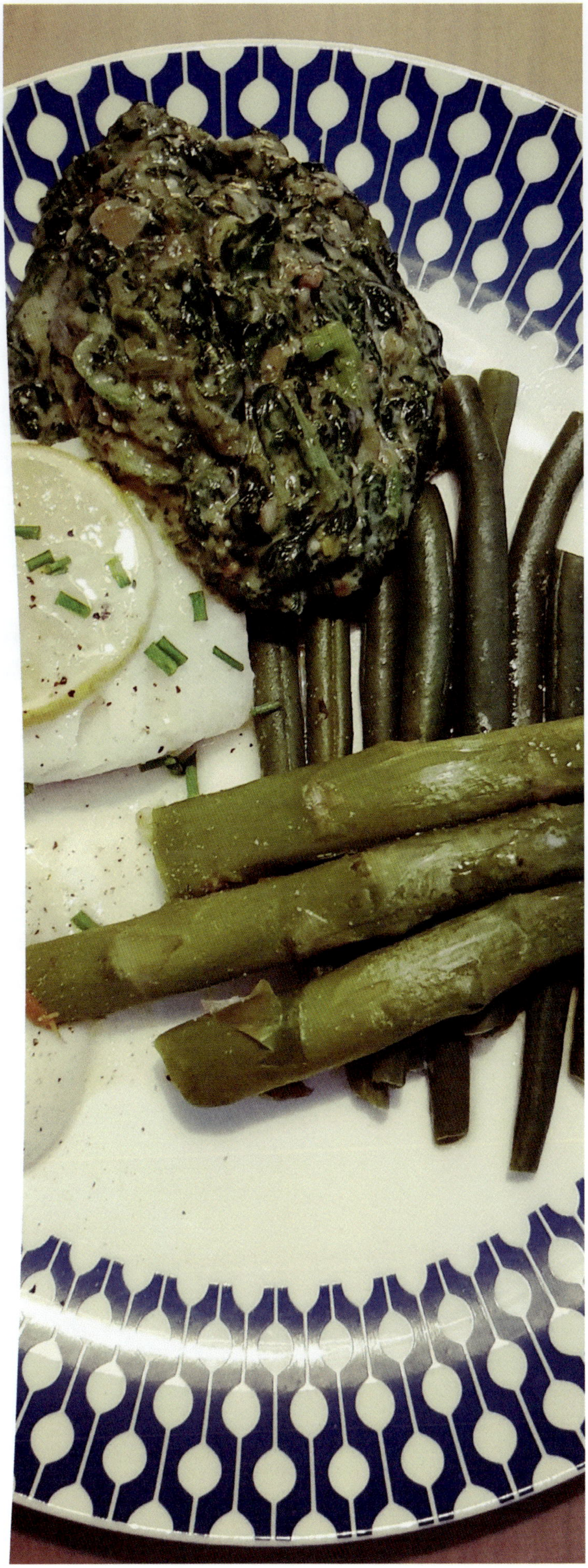

- 6oz Cod fillet, baked in foil with lemon slices, salt and 1 tsp butter
- 3 Spears Asparagus
- 2 tbsp Creamed Spinach
- ½ Cup Green Beans

Carbs 8g
Fat 19g
Protein 38g

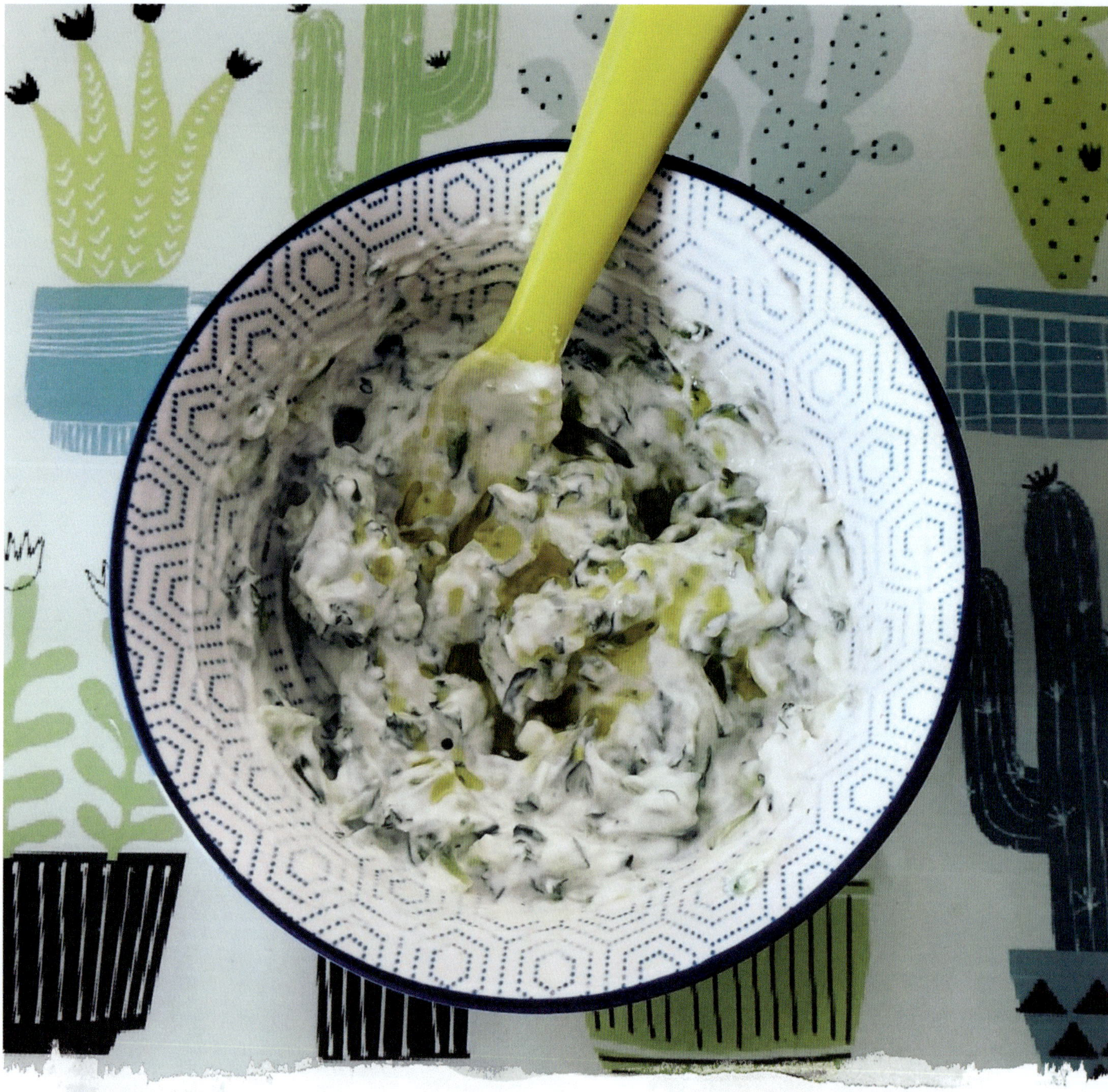

Santorini Tzatziki Dip

- 2 Tbsp full fat Greek yoghurt
- 1/3 cucumber, finely shredded
- 1 Tbsp olive oil
- Salt and pepper
- 1 Tbsp fresh mint

Carbs 6g
Fat 24g
Protein 4g

Squeeze any moisture from the cucumber with a kitchen towel. Combine the yoghurt, mint and garlic, then add the cucumber. Drizzle the oil over the top. Serve with Greek lamb for an incredible meal!

Pecan Cheesecake

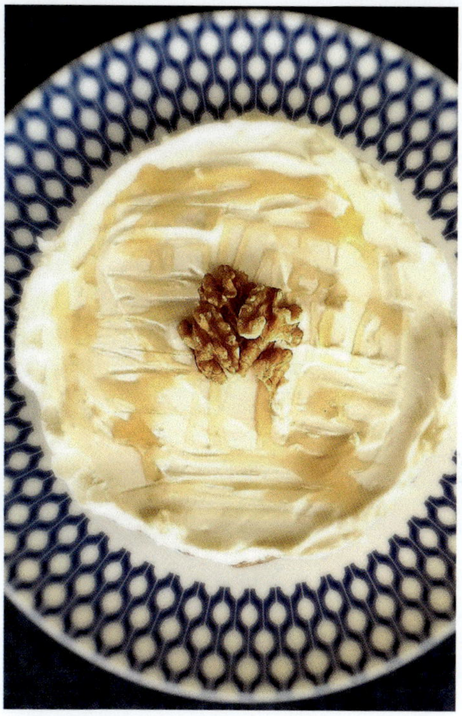

Base

- 2 cups pecans
- 6 tablespoons butter unsalted
- 1 teaspoon vanilla extract
- 1/4 cup erythritol low carb sweetener

Filling

- 16 oz cream cheese softened
- 1 1/4 cup heavy cream
- 1/4 cup erythritol low carb sweetener
- 1 teaspoon vanilla

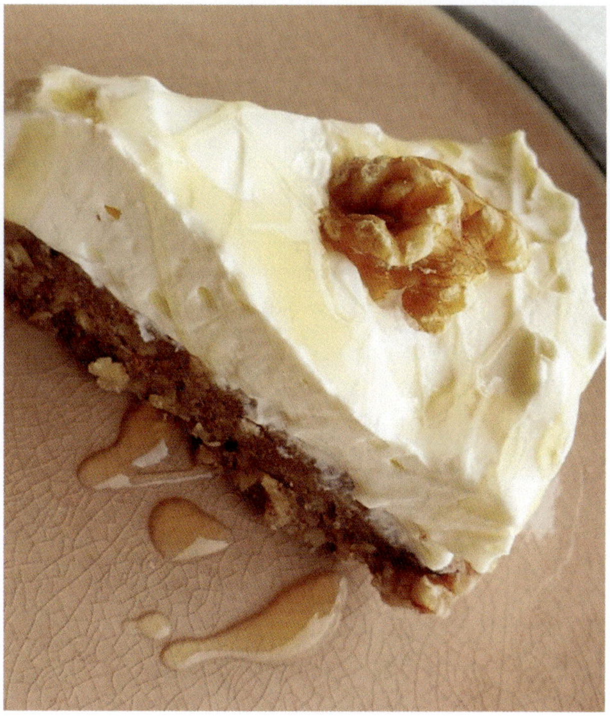

Place pecans in a food processor and blitz until ground. Be careful not to over process as you will end up with butter.

In a bowl, mix the ground pecans, butter, erythritol and vanilla.

Line a spring-form 8-inch cake tin with parchment paper.

Spoon the base mixture into the cake tin and spread evenly, pressing down so the base is firm. Place in the fridge to firm whilst you make the filling

Filling

Place cream cheese in a bowl and whisk until smooth.

Add the cream, erythritol and vanilla and continue to whisk until the mixture is smooth, thick and creamy.

Spoon the mixture over the base evenly.

Carbs 5g

Fat 27g

Protein 8g

High/Moderate Carb Days

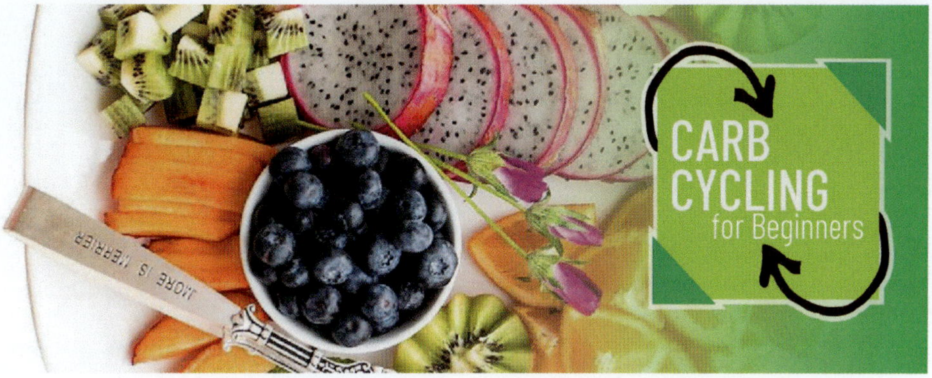

Moderate Carb Day

FOR me, I find moderate day the trickiest. I work easier with extremes and this day for me has neither extremes of carbs or fat, rather a middle ground in all areas.

The most important thing is to really stick to the grams given on these days to make sure it does its job before you go head first into high carb day.

You can also do some exercise on this day! Nothing too crazy or you will end up hungry. Save the full workout for your high carb days. I recommend light weights, relaxed swimming, walking, yoga, pilates or a steady cycle ride.

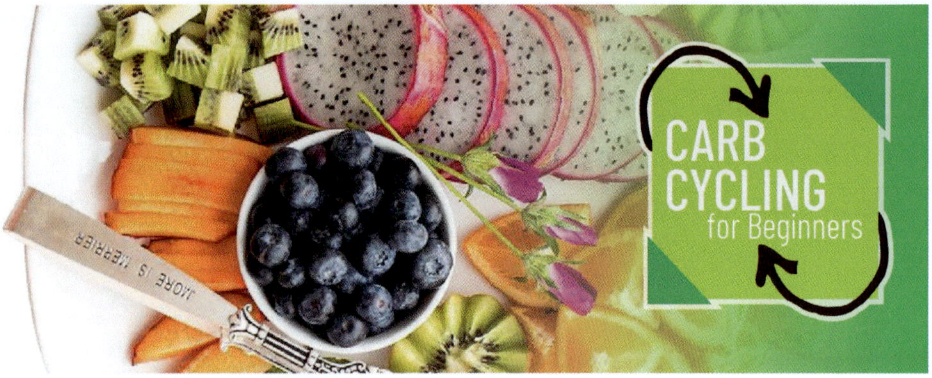

High Carb Day

FOR some, the holy grail of the week. For others, a day where you feel hungrier than all the other days and maybe even slightly bloated.

For those who enjoy exercise, this is your day to go for it, no limits. Push your heart rate and feed your body with the carbs it needs.

Your body will have a shock, but a very good one! A lot of clients report seeing their best loss on the scales the morning after high carb day.

Remember, feed with good carbs. Veggies, fruit, whole wheat bread, rice pasta, sweet potato etc. complex carbs. THIS IS NOT AN EXCUSE TO DRINK FULL FAT COKE!

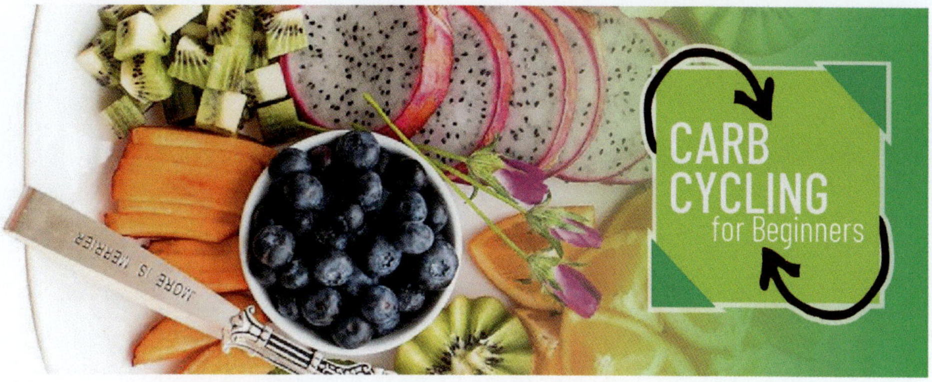

High Carb Day

Foods to eat alongside
meat fish and eggs

- Bananas
- Oranges
- Apples
- Mango
- Pineapple
- Sweet potato
- Plantains
- Beans
- Whole wheat Rice
- Whole wheat Pasta
- Whole wheat Bread
- Oatmeal
- Blueberries
- Low fat Greek Yoghurt
- Dried fruit

Breakfast

I actually find high carb day breakfast quite challenging sometimes as my palette seems to prefer the high fat foods when I wake up!

Eggs feature again, though less heavily, but now is the time for those oats to make an appearance!

Toast is an option of course but I couldn't bring myself to do a recipe page just for that.... Just be sure to have it without butter!

The Perfect Brunch

- 2 eggs, poached
- ½ avocado, mashed with lemon juice, salt and pepper
- 2 Slices whole wheat toast

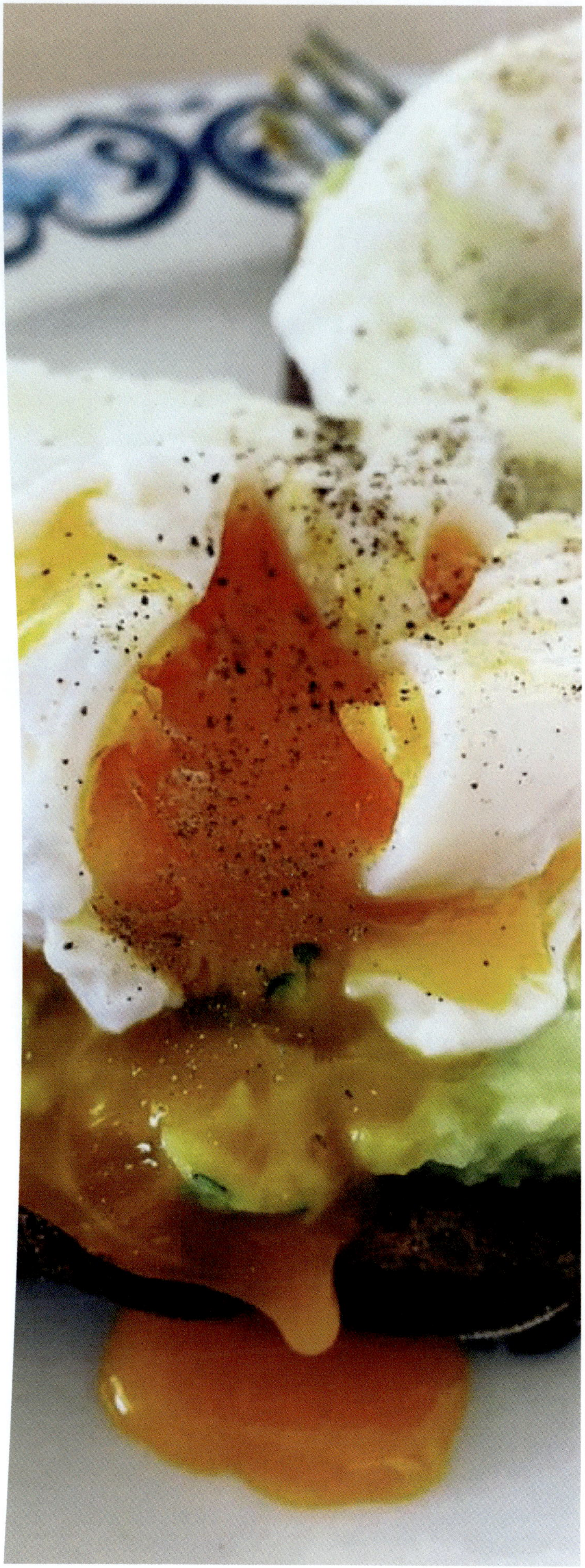

Carbs 32g
Fat 22g
Protein 20g

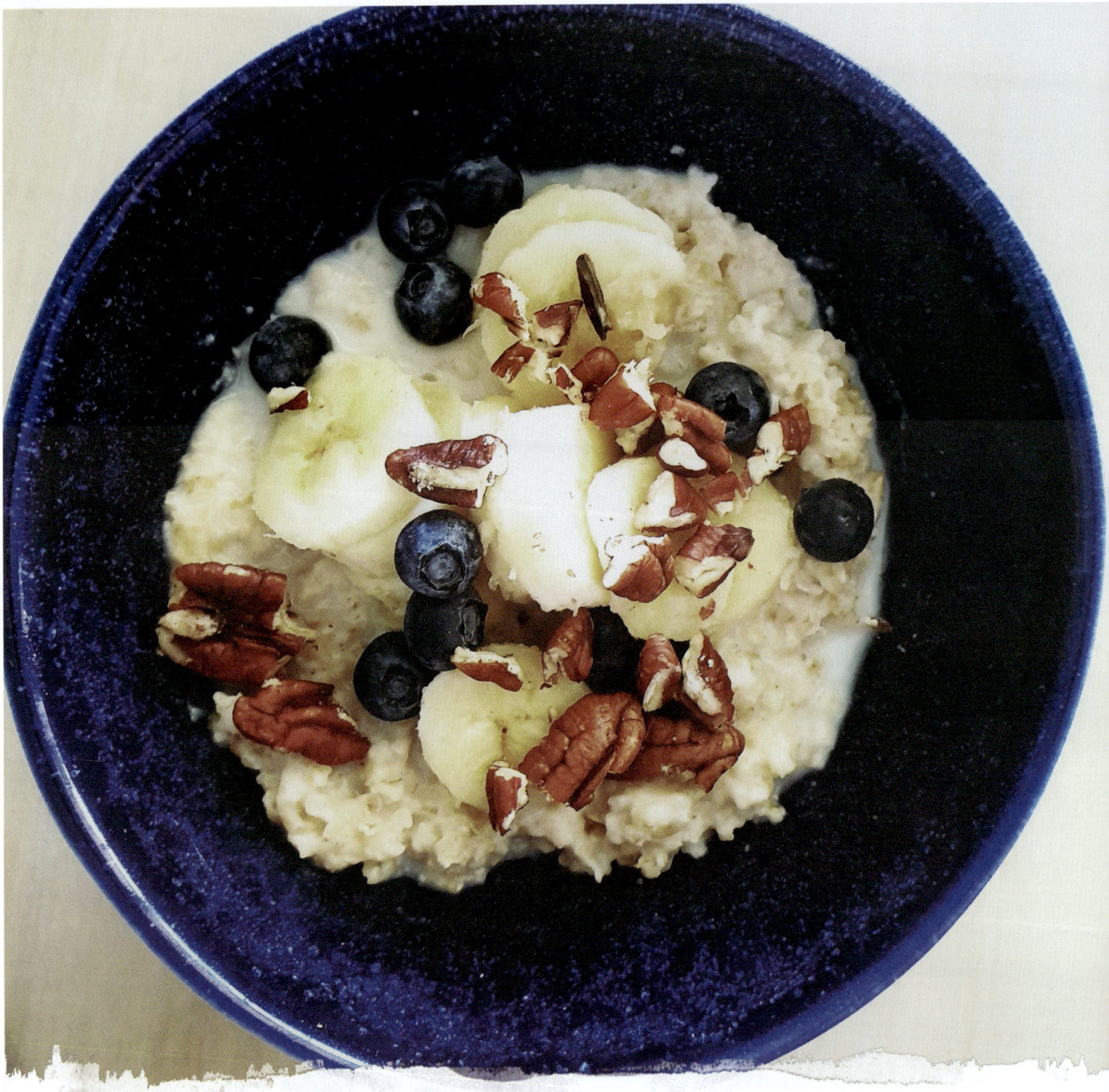

Warming Banana Honey Oats

- 1 Banana
- 1 Tsp Honey
- 1 tbsp blueberries
- 200ml Unsweetened Almond Milk
- ½ cup oats
- 3 Pecan Halves

Carbs 86g
Fat 19g
Protein 17g

Super Green Smoothie

- 1 Green Apple
- 10 Green Grapes
- 50g Baby Spinach
- 5 fresh mint leaves
- ½ Ripe Avocado
- 1 scoop flavorless protein
- 1 tsp fresh ginger

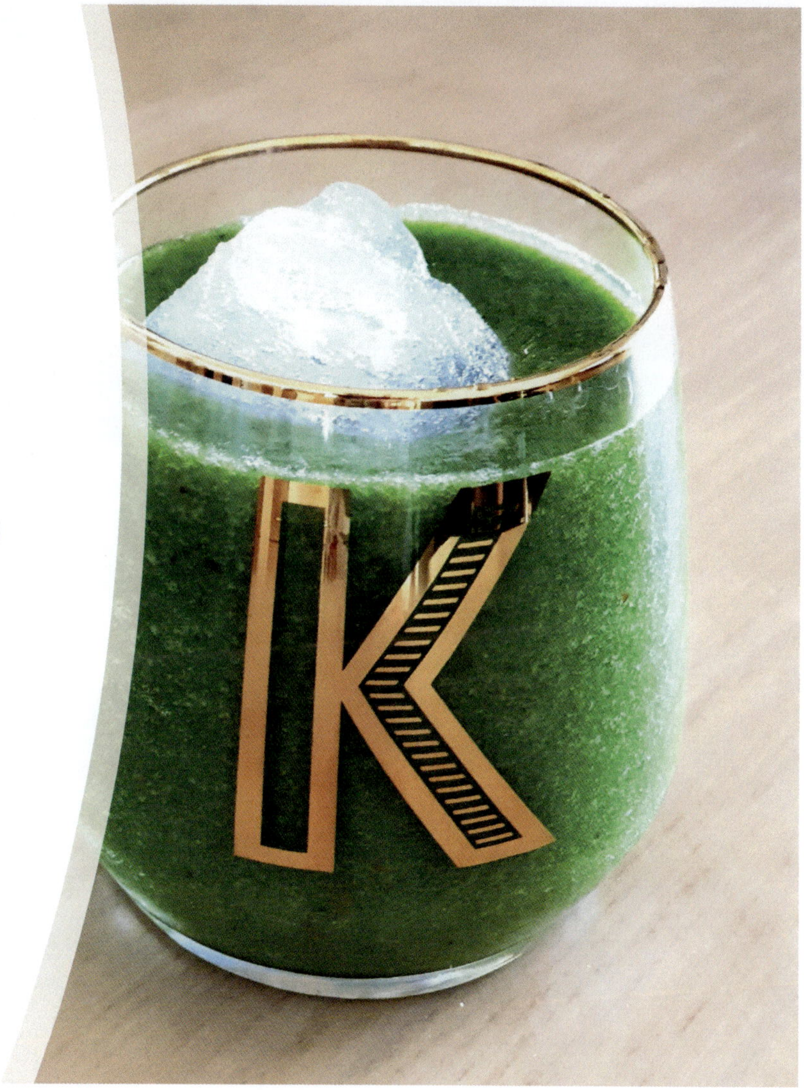

Carbs 49.9g
Fat 13.4g
Protein 30.5g

Classic Bagels

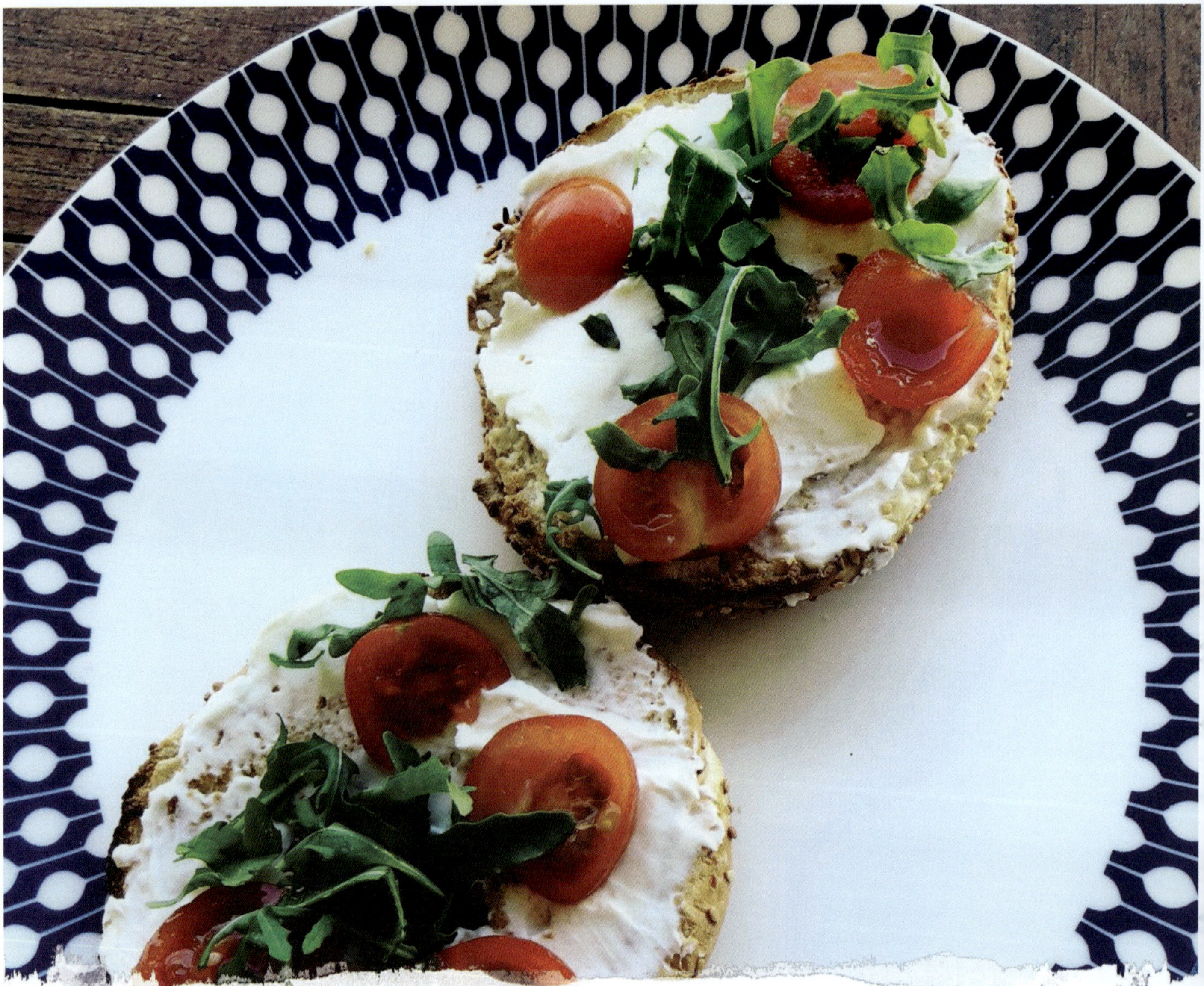

1 x Sesame or Everything Bagel

30g Low Fat Cream Cheese

4 Cherry Tomatoes

Rocket/Arugula

Seriously simple, toast the bagels, spread on the cream cheese, halve the tomatoes and garnish with the Rocket!

Carbs 34.2g, Fat 3.7g, Protein 9.9g

Lunch

It is important on high carb day to get as many carbs in as you can, without leaving it all for your evening meal.

I have opted for recipes that are higher carbs but not heavy on the stomach, to ensure you are not found asleep at your desk at 3 o'clock in the afternoon!

Carbs do not have to be heavy, there are many cunning ways of eating a lot without weighing you down.

Creamy Celeriac Soup

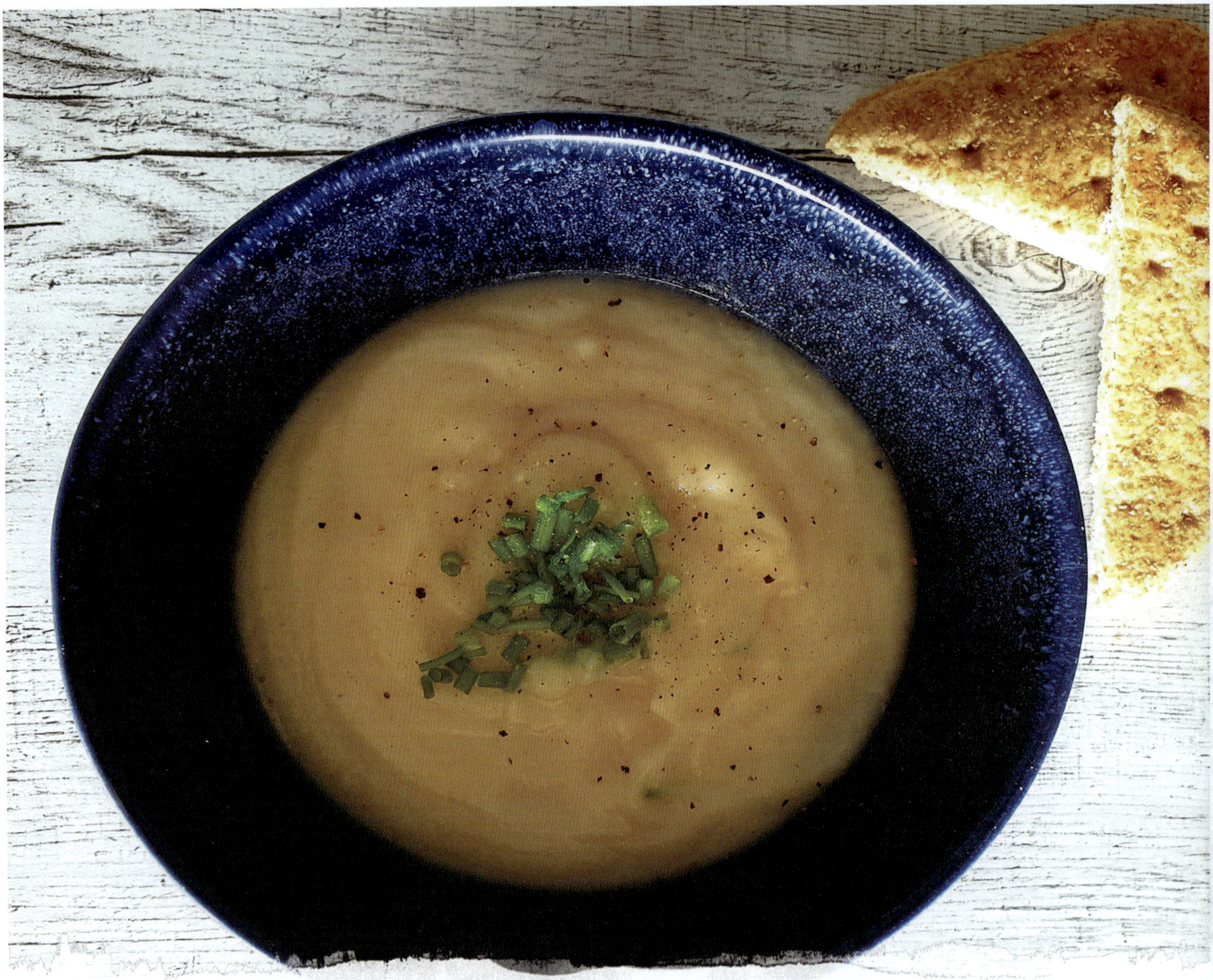

Half a celeriac (Celery root)
1 tbsp low fat cream cheese
Water

Steam the celeriac until soft, add the cheese and blend!
Serve with 1 whole wheat 'thin'

Carbs 30g
Fat 3g
Protein 8g

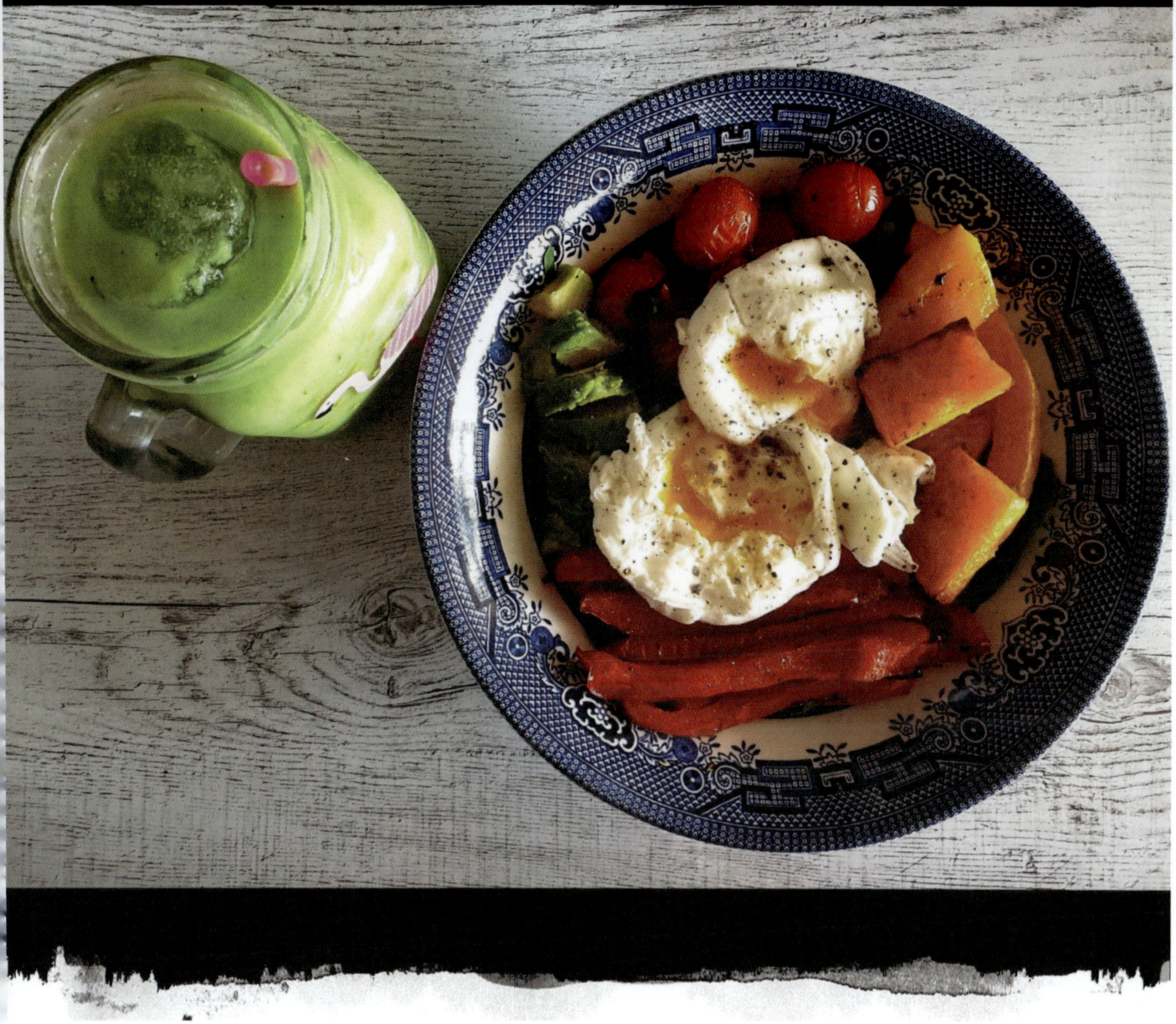

Rainbow Bowl

- 1/3 Cup Roasted Butternut Squash
- ¼ Ripe avocado
- 1 tbsp Baby spinach
- 100g Roasted red peppers
- 5 Whole cherry tomatoes
- 2 Poached eggs

Carbs 22g

Fat 16g

Protein 15g

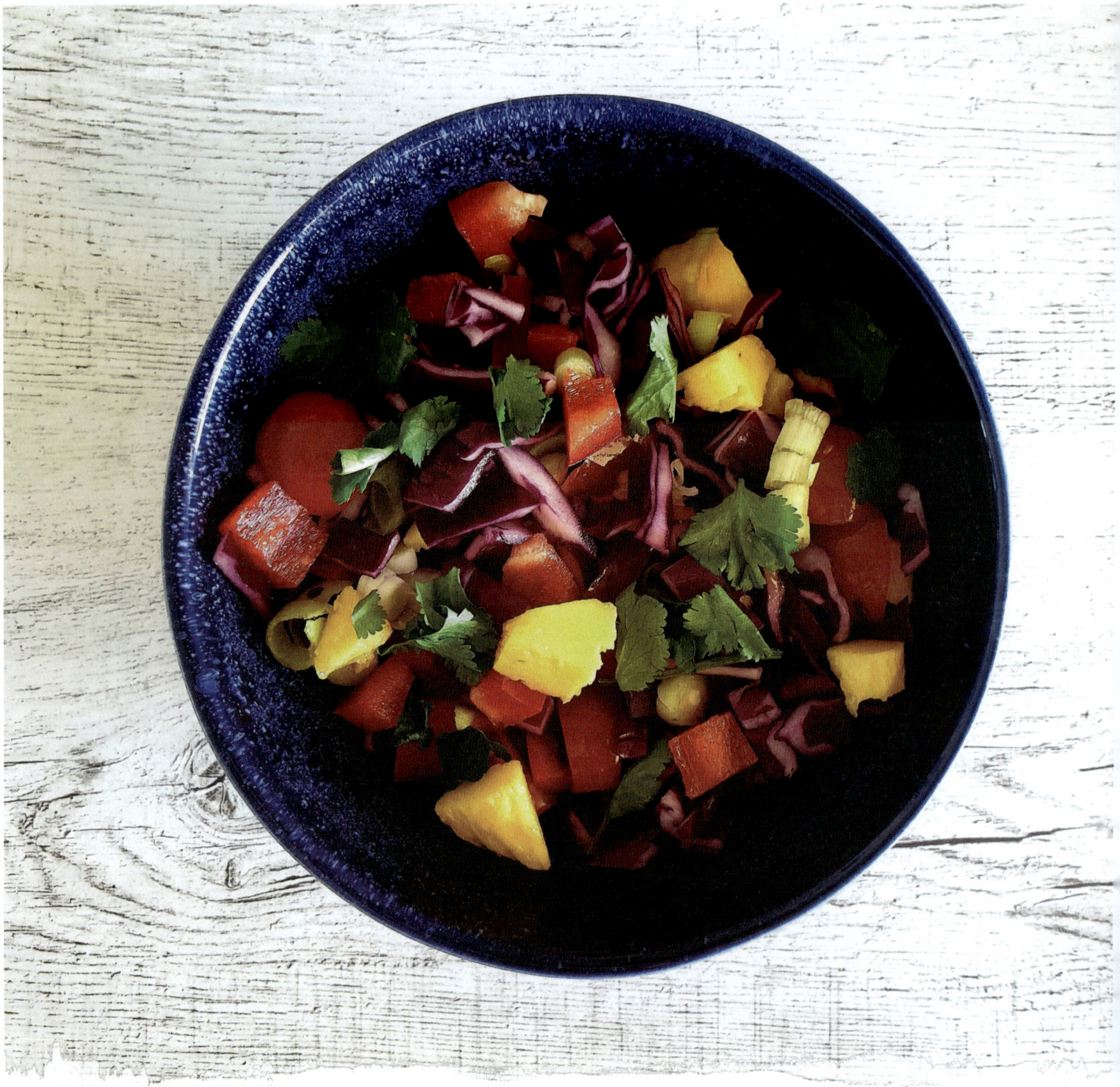

Summer Coleslaw

- 1 Cup red cabbage
- ¼ cup mango
- 5 Cherry tomatoes
- ½ cup red pepper
- 1 Tbsp fresh coriander
- 1 Spring/green onion stalk, chopped small

Carbs 21g
Fat 0g
Protein 3g

Avocado Salsa

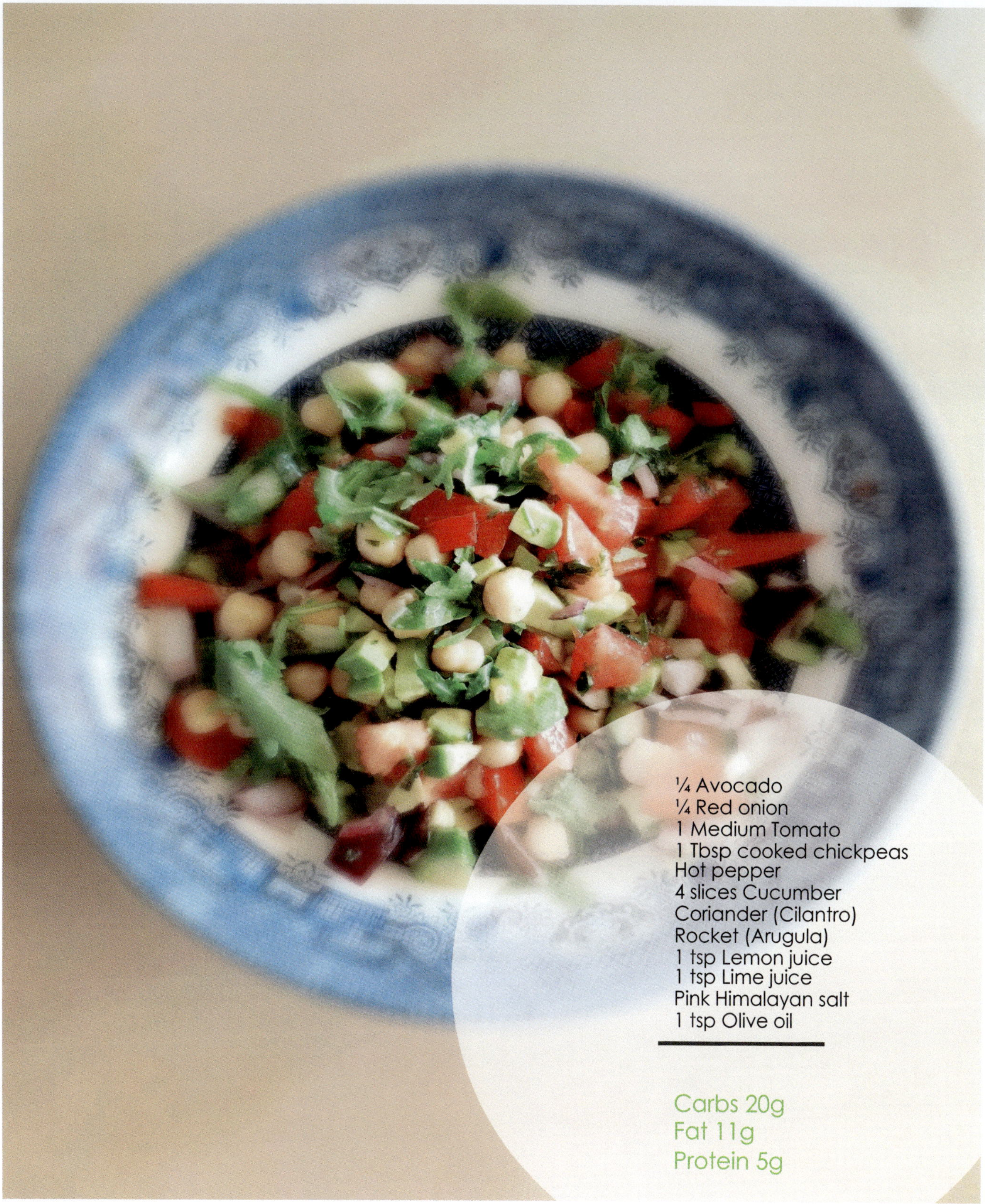

¼ Avocado
¼ Red onion
1 Medium Tomato
1 Tbsp cooked chickpeas
Hot pepper
4 slices Cucumber
Coriander (Cilantro)
Rocket (Arugula)
1 tsp Lemon juice
1 tsp Lime juice
Pink Himalayan salt
1 tsp Olive oil

Carbs 20g
Fat 11g
Protein 5g

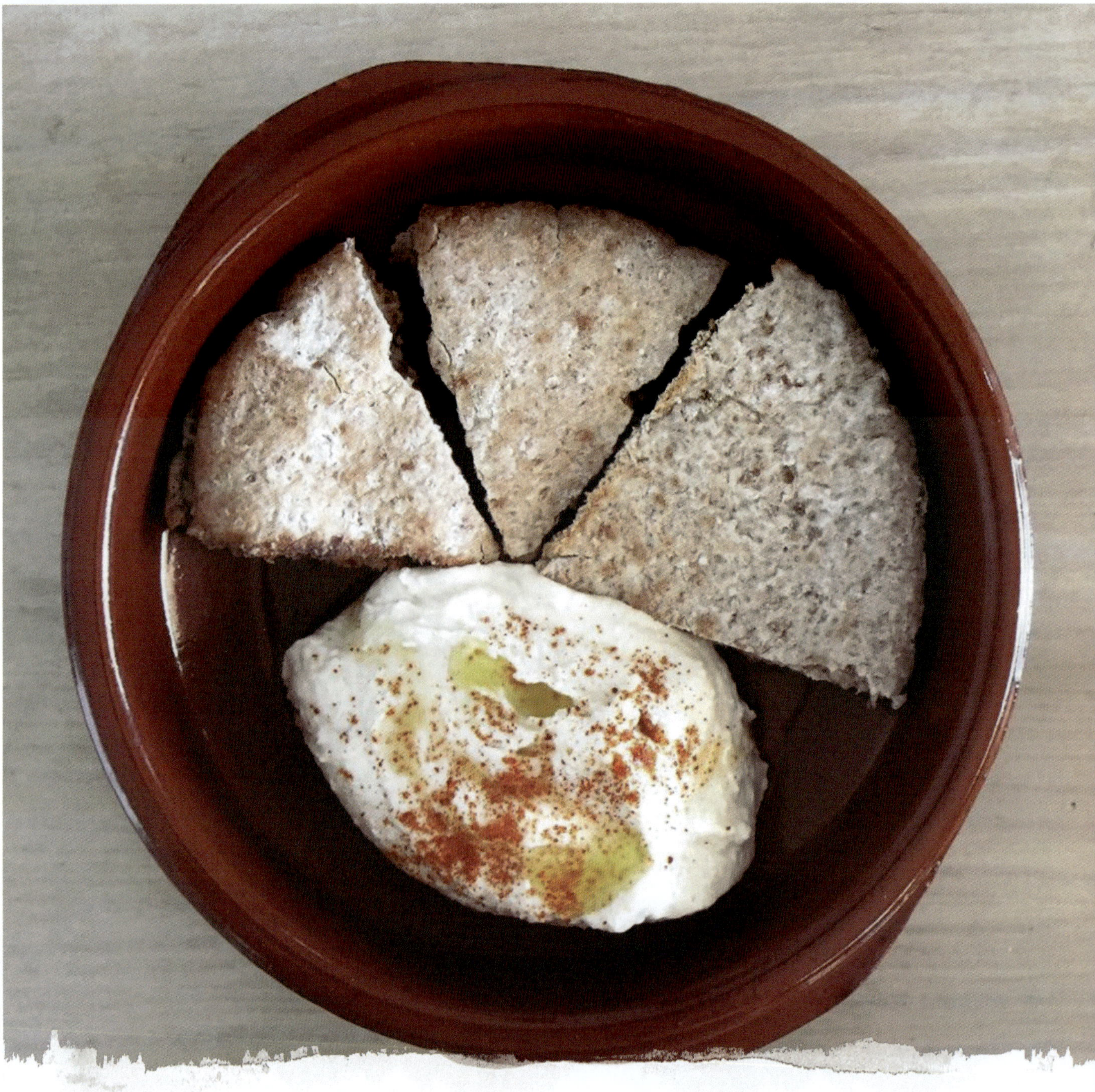

Fresh Houmous

- Half a Canned/Jar Chickpeas
- 2 Tbsp Sesame seeds
- 2 Tbsp Lemon Juice
- 1 Tsp Garlic paste/crushed garlic
- 1 Tbsp Olive oil

Carbs 50g, Fat 30.4g, Protein 23.7g

Add all ingredients to a blender ensuring all chickpeas are pulped. Adjust quantities to reach desired taste.

To serve drizzle olive oil and season with Paprika.

Serve with Toasted whole wheat pitta bread

Dinner

The kids will rejoice at this one – pasta for dinner finally, hooray!

It is a day to eat without guilt, and if you have previously done Keto or a strict low carb diet, you may find high carb dinners a little overwhelming at first, but believe me you will soon get used to it and most of all, enjoy it!

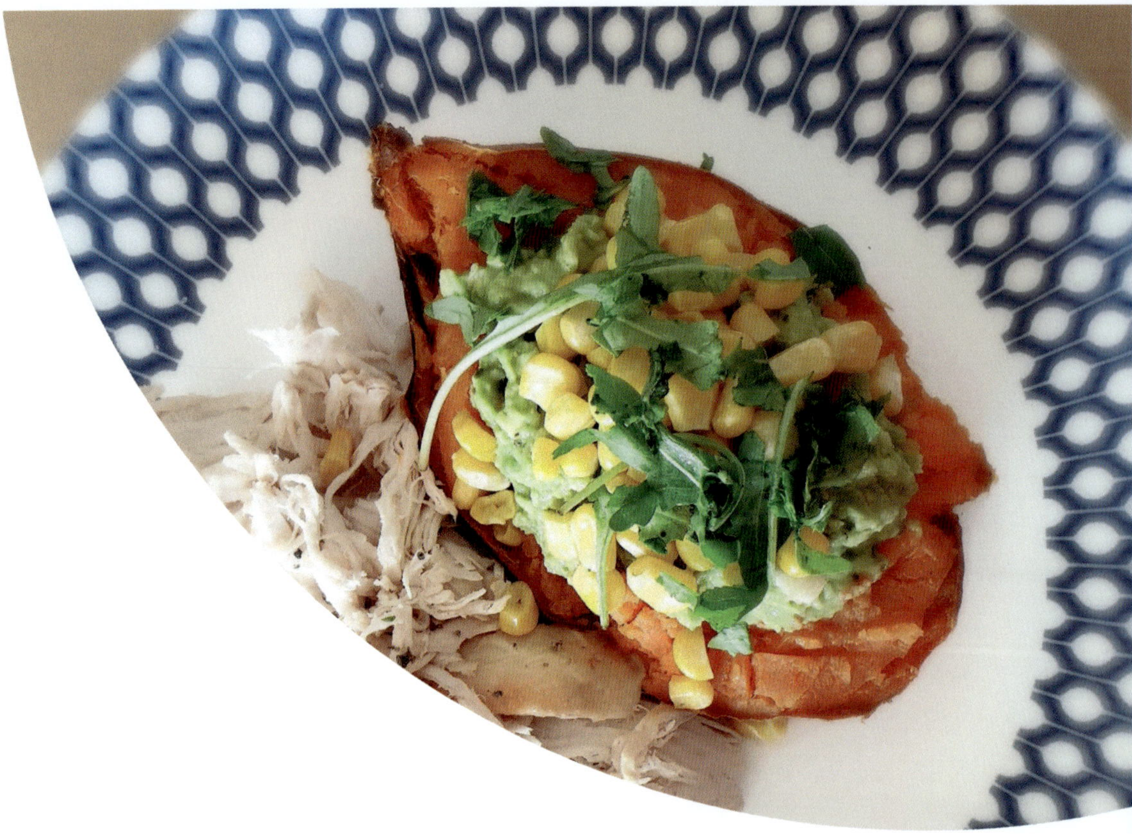

- 1 Medium sweet potato
- 1 small ripe avocado
- 100g Canned sweetcorn
- 1 7oz Roasted chicken breast

Bake the sweet potato until soft with a crispy skin. Mash the avocado and top the potato. Add the sweetcorn and season the chicken breast.

Carbs 57g
Fat 24g
Protein 34g

Avocado Stuffed Sweet Potato with Roast Chicken

Mild Spiced Warming Lentils

Serves 3

1 cup brown lentils
1 cup Butternut Squash, diced
1 cup cooked chickpeas
1 tbsp cumin
1 clove garlic
1 cup frozen creamed
Spinach
¼ cup red onion
Salt and pepper
Handful fresh coriander
1 tsp low fat yoghurt, to serve

Put all ingredients except coriander and yoghurt in a large pan, with 300ml water and simmer, adding more water as the lentils absorb it, until the lentils are soft.

Garnish with the yoghurt and small piece of coriander

Carbs 73g, Fat 10g, Protein 23g

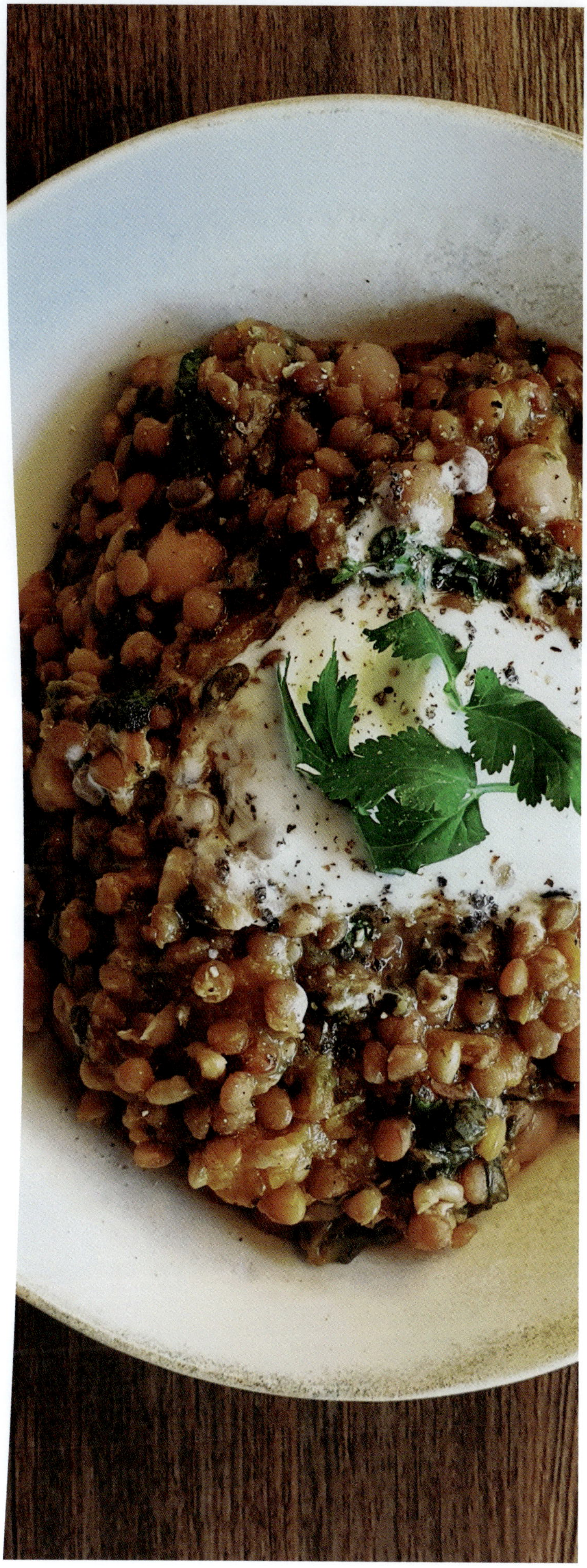

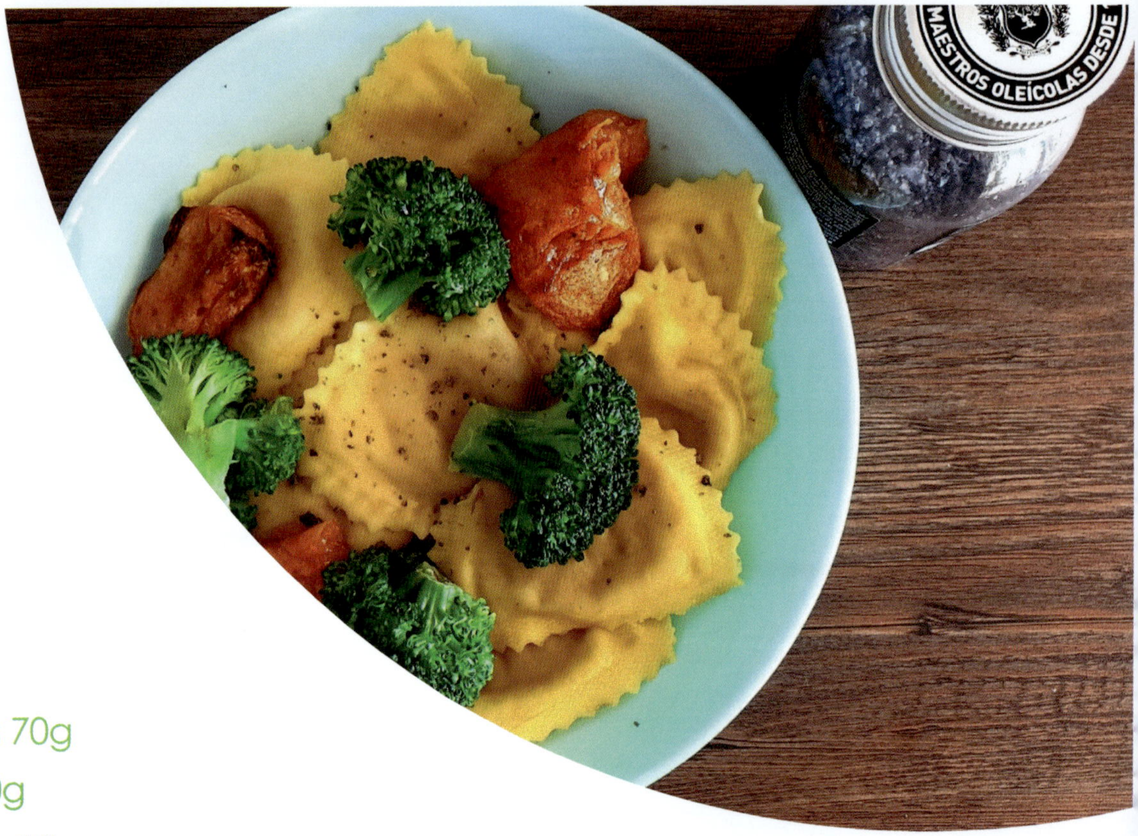

Carbs 70g

Fat 20g

Protein15g

- 100g Butternut Squash tortellini
- 1 Cup Roasted Butternut squash
- 100g Broccoli, steamed

Squash Tortellini

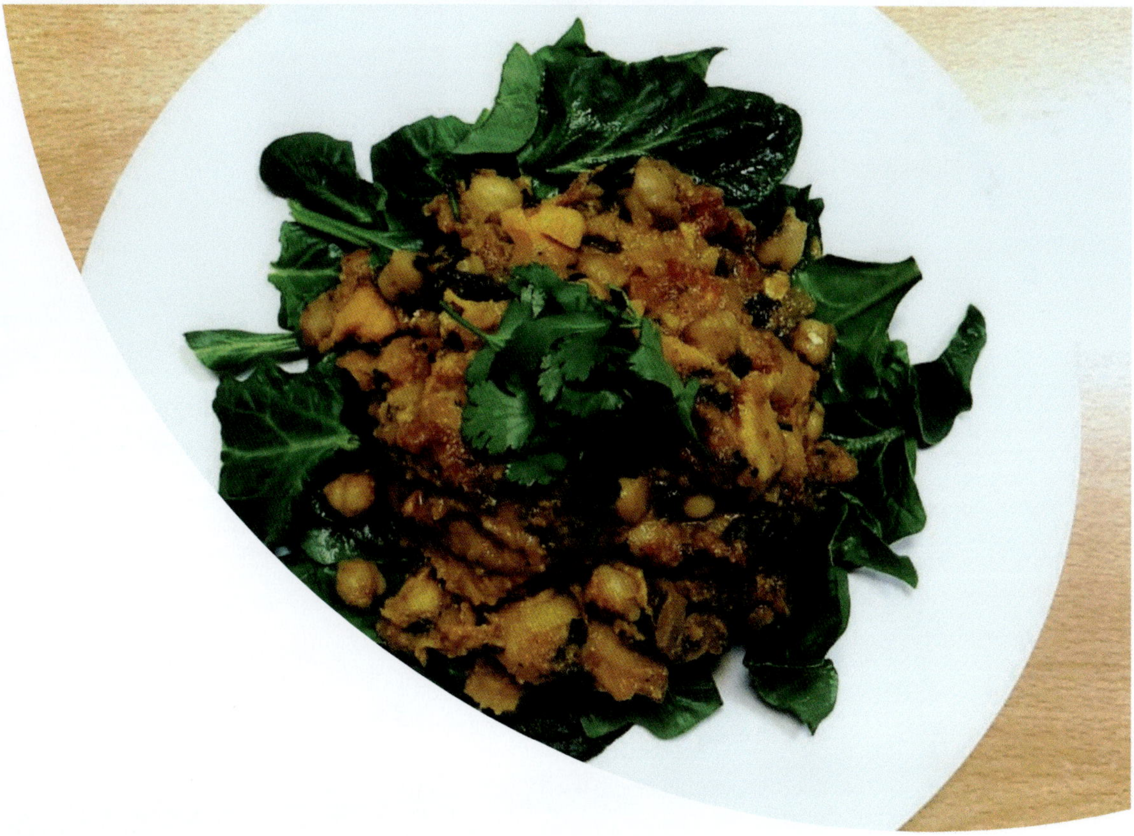

Serves 4

- 2 Medium sweet potato
- 1 Can cooked chickpeas
- 1 Can chopped tomatoes
- 4oz Low fat coconut milk
- 2oz Creamed spinach
- 1 Tbsp curry powder
- 1 Tsp turmeric
- 1 clove garlic, minced

Put all ingredients into a large cooking pot or slow cooker,and cook for 3 hours on low.

Carbs 46g
Fat 11g
Protein 14g

Sweet Potato and Chickpea Curry

Autumn Risotto

- 1.1 litres stock (chicken, fish, vegetable)
- 1 large onion
- 2 cloves of garlic
- ½ a head of celery
- 2 tablespoons olive oil
- unsalted butter
- 400 g risotto rice
- 2 wine glasses of dry white vermouth or dry white wine
- ½ cup roasted squash
- ½ cup fried mushrooms

Method

- Heat the stock. Peel and finely chop the onion and garlic, trim and finely chop celery
- In a separate pan, heat the oil and 1 small knob of butter over a low heat, add the onions, garlic and celery, and fry gently for 15 minutes, or until softened but not coloured.
- Add the rice and turn up the heat – the rice will now begin to lightly fry, so keep stirring it. After 1 minute it will look slightly translucent. Add the vermouth or wine and keep stirring. Any harsh alcohol flavours will evaporate and leave the rice with a tasty essence.
- Once the wine has cooked into the rice, add your first ladle of hot stock and a pinch of sea salt. Turn the heat down to a simmer so the rice doesn't cook too quickly on the outside.
- Keep adding ladlefuls of stock, stirring and almost massaging the creamy starch out of the rice, allowing each ladleful to be absorbed before adding the next. This will take around 15 minutes. Taste the rice, is it cooked? Carry on adding stock until the rice is soft but with a slight bite. Don't forget to check the seasoning carefully. If you run out of stock before the rice is cooked, add some boiling water.
- Remove from the heat, add 1 knob of butter, then stir well.
- Place a lid on the pan and allow to sit for 2 minutes – this is the most important part of making the perfect risotto, as this is when it becomes outrageously creamy and oozy like it should be. Eat it as soon as possible, while the risotto retains its beautiful texture.

Carbs 59g

Fat 10g

Protein 15.1g

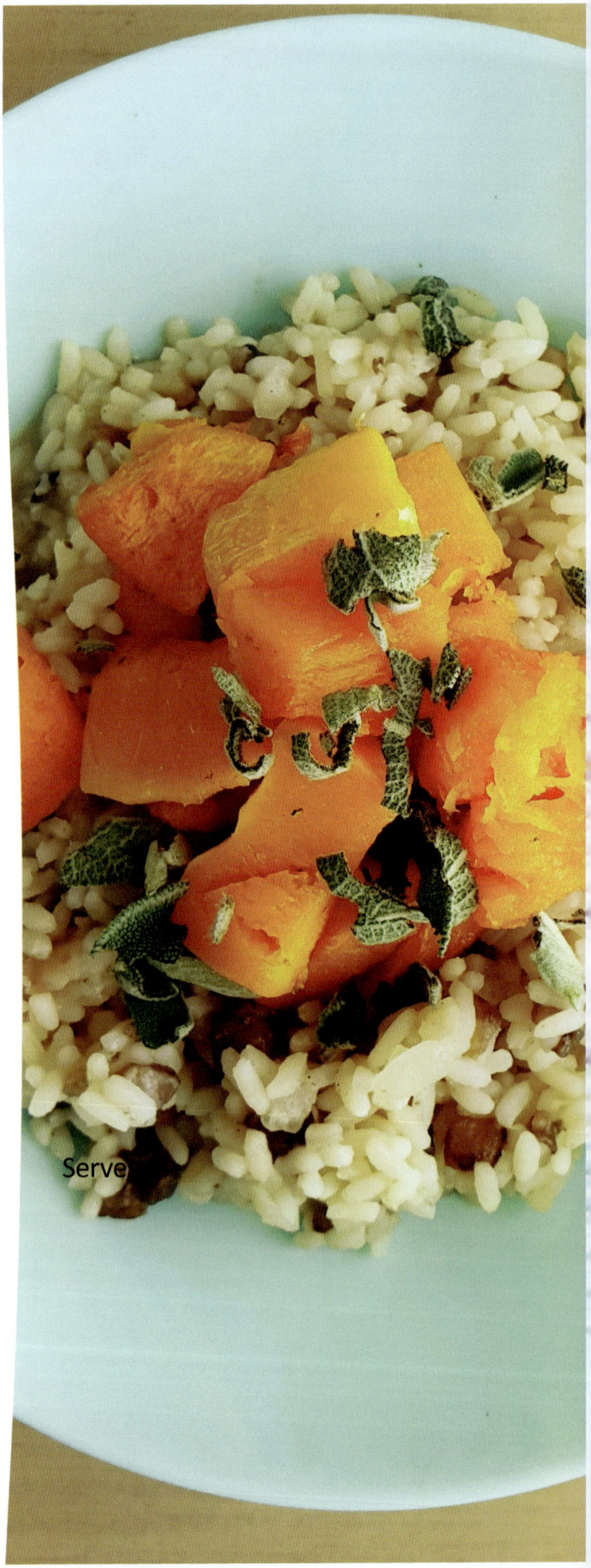

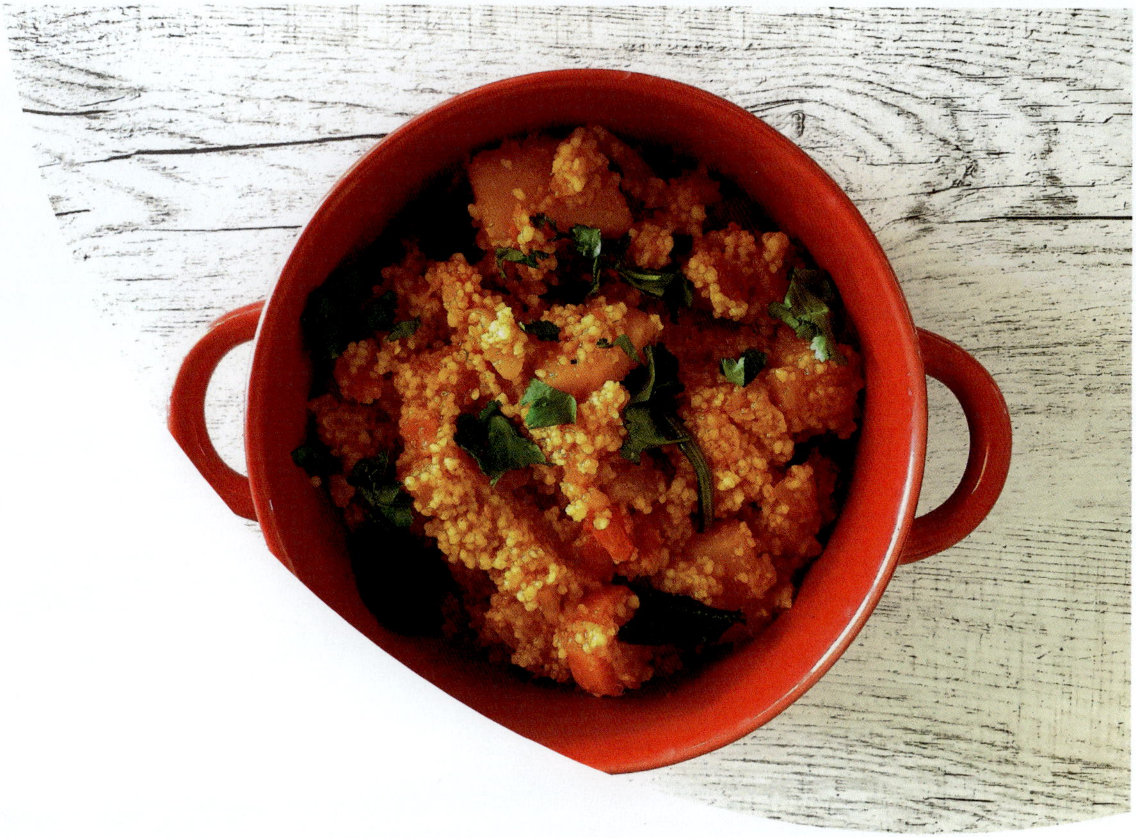

Moroccan Meat Free Tagine

Serves 4

- 2 Whole carrots, chopped
- 1 Cup butternut squash, chopped
- ½ White onion, chopped
- 3 Large garlic cloves, minced
- 1 Cup uncooked couscous
- 2 Tbsp olive oil
- 1 ½ Tbsp paprika
- 1 ½ tsp curry powder
- 2 Stalks celery
- ¼ Tsp cinnamon
- Salt and pepper

Carbs 34g
Fat 10g
Protein 6g

Soften the squash, carrots, onion and celery in the olive oil.

Add the garlic, paprika, cinnamon and curry powder and stir in briefly.

Add the canned tomatoes and cous cous, keep on a very low heat and add 1 cup of water. Cook for one hour, topping up the water.

Garnish with fresh coriander.

Coconut Curry with Rice

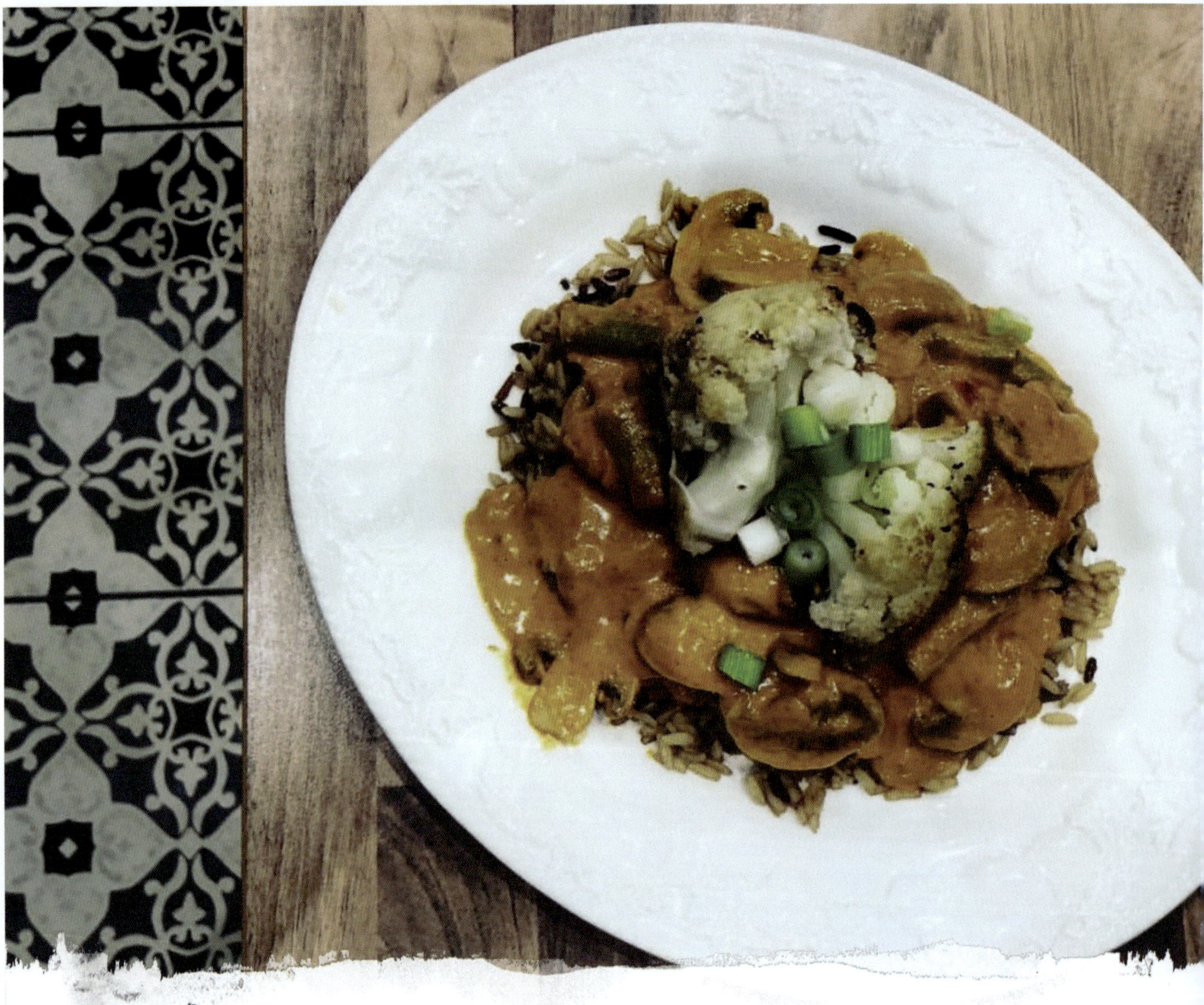

- 1 Cup Cauliflower
- 100ml Low Fat Coconut milk
- 200g Canned Tomatoes
- 2 Tbsp Curry Powder
- 1 Tbsp Cumin
- 50g Chestnut Mushrooms
- 1 Fresh Chili, de-seeded
- 50g Brown rice

The beauty of this dish is that it can all be thrown into the slow cooker on low for over 4 hours. Slice the mushrooms, grill the cauliflower first to give an extra flavor, and leave to simmer away, enjoying the incredible smell!

If you need more protein you can always add chicken/beef/turkey.

Carbs 56g, Fat 10g, Protein 11.2g

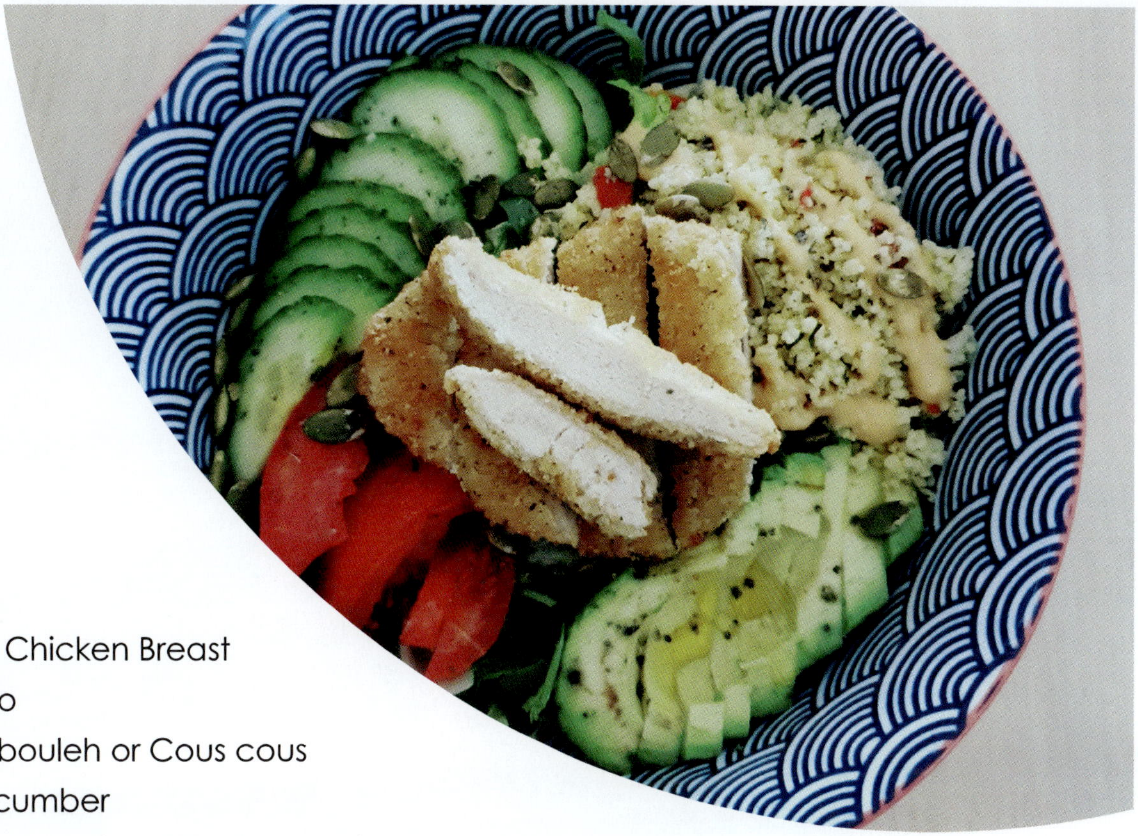

- 1 Breaded Chicken Breast
- ½ Avocado
- 1 Tbsp Tabbouleh or Cous cous
- ¼ Cup Cucumber
- 1 Tomato
- 1 Cup Lettuce
- 1 tsp Olive oil

Carbs 23g
Fat 20g
Protein 23g

Crispy Chicken and Tabbouleh Poke Bowl

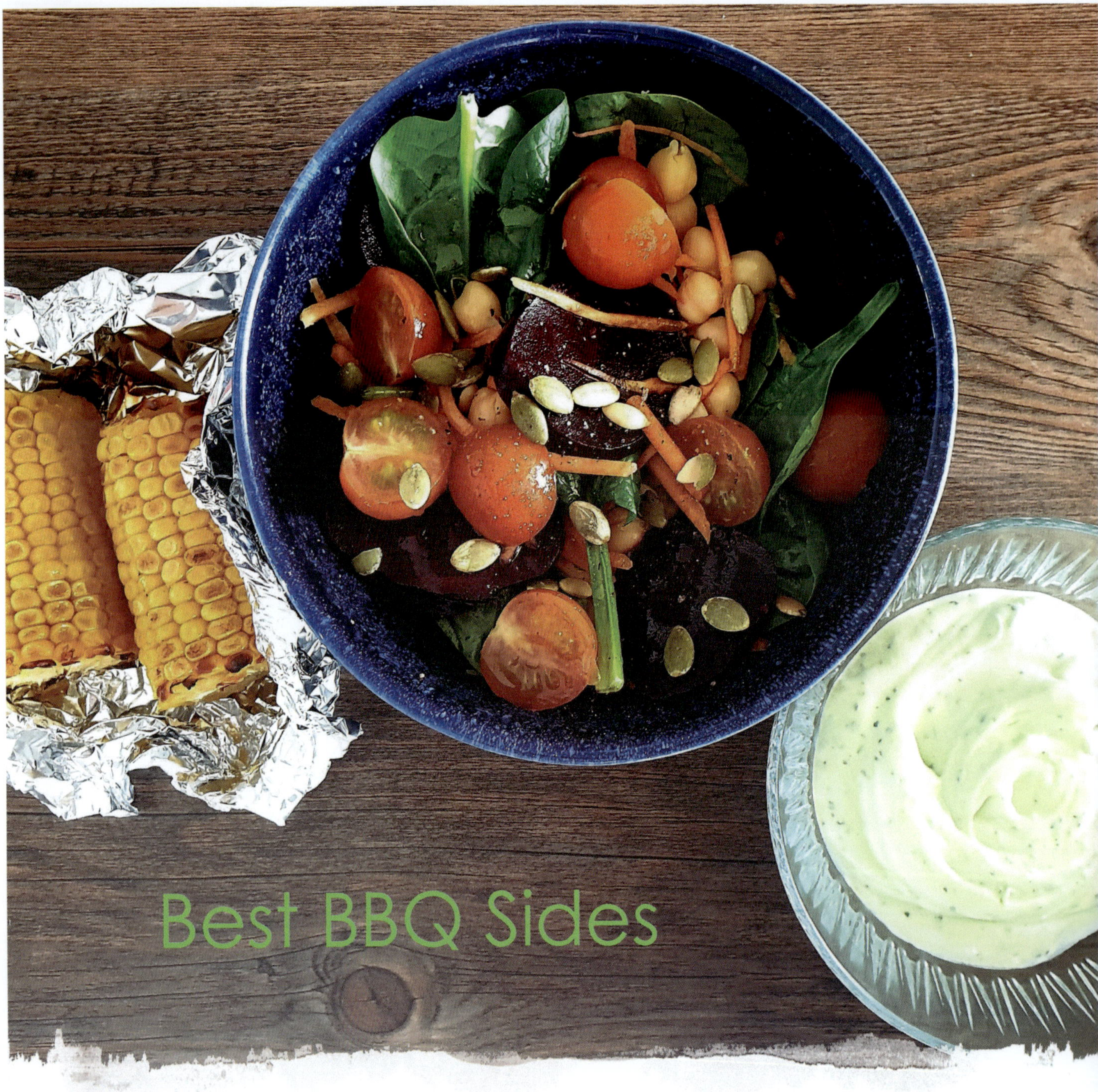

Best BBQ Sides

- 2 Tbsp cooked chickpeas
- 5 Cherry tomatoes
- 1 Cup baby spinach
- 1 Corn on the cob, grilled
- 25g Grated carrot
- ½ whole small cooked beetroot
- ¼ Ripe avocado

Add your favorite low fat salad dressing!

Carbs 63g
Fat 9g
Protein 13g

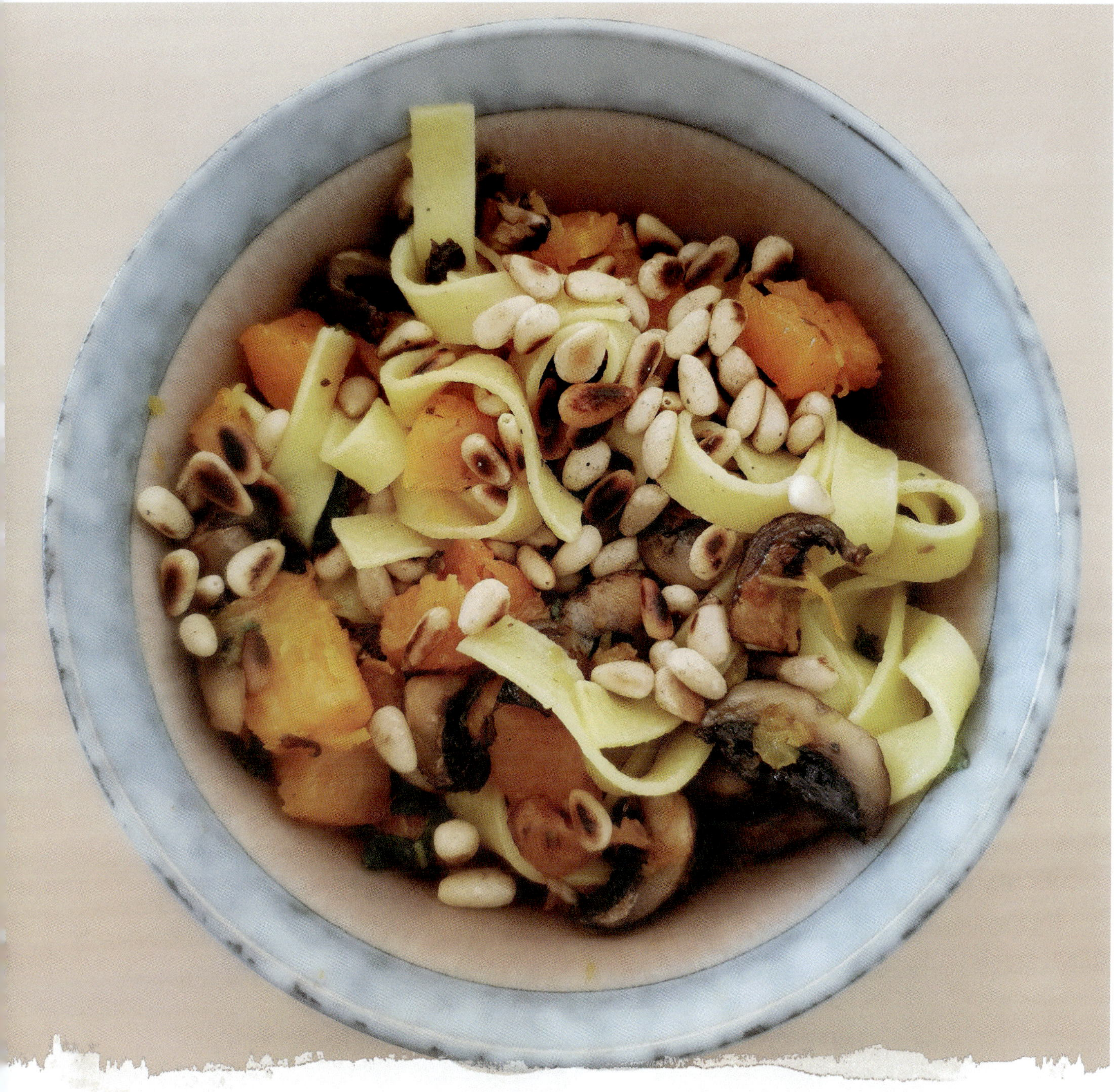

Mushroom Sage and Squash Tagliatelle

- 100g fresh tagliatelle, boiled
- ½ cup mushrooms, fried in 1 tsp oil
- 1 cup roasted butternut squash
- 1/2 tbsp pine nuts, gently toasted

Carbs 62g

Fat 13g

Protein 9g

Creamy Veggie Curry

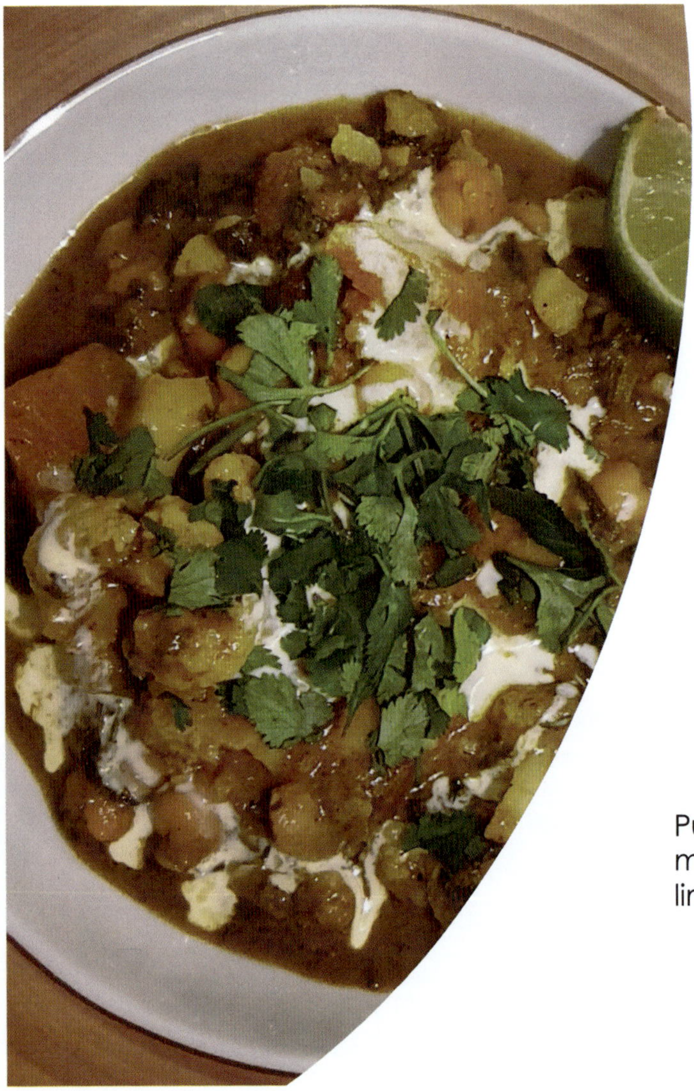

Serves 2

- 1 cup Butternut squash
- 4 tbsp Creamed Chickpeas
- Low fat Coconut milk, skim the cream from the top of the tin and use about 1/3 of the liquid
- 1 cup Cauliflower
- Turmeric
- Ginger
- Coriander (stalks only, leaves for garnish)
- 2 fresh chillies
- 2 cloves garlic
- Cayenne pepper
- Curry powder
- Cumin
- 1 tbsp of tomato puree

Put the entire contents into a slow cooker for minimum 3 hours on high, and garnish with lime wedges and coriander leaves

Carbs 43g, Fat 21g, Protein 12g

Meal Planning

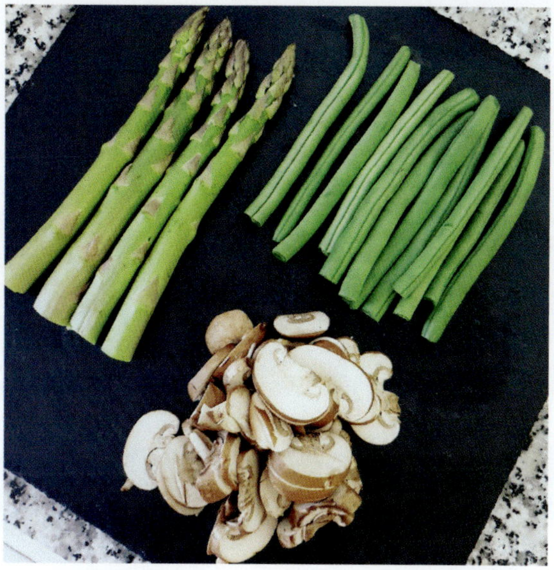

Be sure to plan out your week in advance, to ensure you won't get caught out!

Apps such as MyFitnessPal and Carb Manager are great to be able to input your macros and plan your food, so that you can see where any gaps may arise, or days which need more work. If you do this, you are much more likely to succeed with hitting those numbers!

Decide which day will be lows, moderate and highs! Take into account any social events if you know you are going to be needing the weekend to have a high day, etc.

Be sure to divide your day equally especially if your carb target is super high on high days. Once you divide it into 3 meals, you'll be surprised how easy it is to hit that goal.

I have added a 7-day template to get you started, simply choose the meal from the book, and add in the macros, to help you reach your custom goal! (If you don't have targets, consider using Kate's private coaching tool!)

Meal Planner

	Macros		
	Carbs	Fat	Protein
Breakfast			
Lunch			
Dinner			

Meal Planner

	Macros		
	Carbs	Fat	Protein
Breakfast			
Lunch			
Dinner			

Meal Planner

	Macros		
	Carbs	Fat	Protein
Breakfast			
Lunch			
Dinner			

Meal Planner

Macros

	Carbs	Fat	Protein
Breakfast			
Lunch			
Dinner			

Meal Planner

	Macros		
	Carbs	Fat	Protein
Breakfast			
Lunch			
Dinner			

Meal Planner

	Macros		
	Carbs	Fat	Protein
Breakfast			
Lunch			
Dinner			

Meal Planner

	Macros		
	Carbs	Fat	Protein
Breakfast			
Lunch			
Dinner			

Notes/Meal Ideas

Notes/Meal Ideas

Weight Conversions

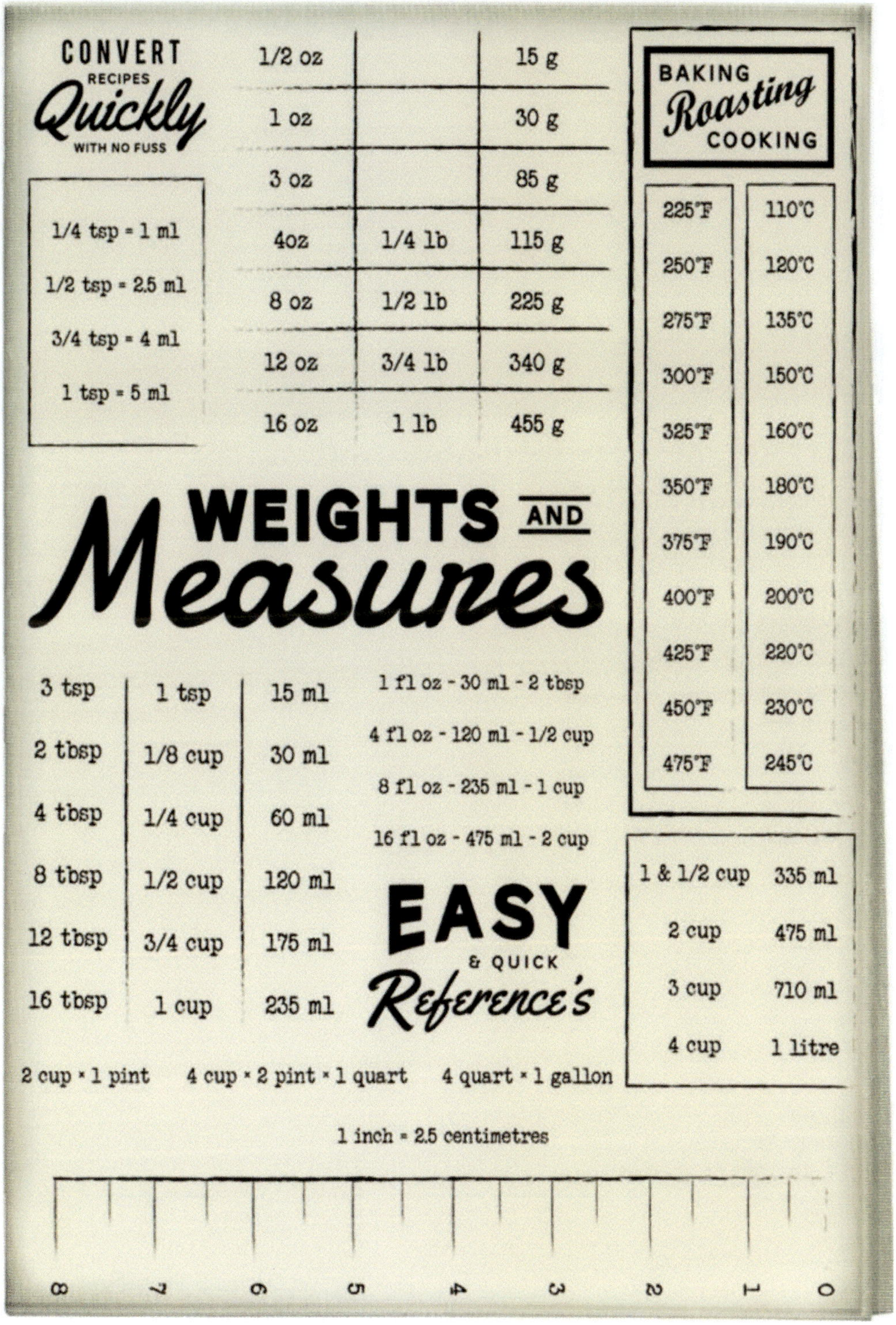

CONVERT RECIPES *Quickly* WITH NO FUSS

1/2 oz		15 g
1 oz		30 g
3 oz		85 g
4oz	1/4 lb	115 g
8 oz	1/2 lb	225 g
12 oz	3/4 lb	340 g
16 oz	1 lb	455 g

1/4 tsp = 1 ml
1/2 tsp = 2.5 ml
3/4 tsp = 4 ml
1 tsp = 5 ml

BAKING *Roasting* COOKING

225°F	110°C
250°F	120°C
275°F	135°C
300°F	150°C
325°F	160°C
350°F	180°C
375°F	190°C
400°F	200°C
425°F	220°C
450°F	230°C
475°F	245°C

WEIGHTS AND *Measures*

3 tsp	1 tsp	15 ml
2 tbsp	1/8 cup	30 ml
4 tbsp	1/4 cup	60 ml
8 tbsp	1/2 cup	120 ml
12 tbsp	3/4 cup	175 ml
16 tbsp	1 cup	235 ml

1 fl oz - 30 ml - 2 tbsp
4 fl oz - 120 ml - 1/2 cup
8 fl oz - 235 ml - 1 cup
16 fl oz - 475 ml - 2 cup

EASY & QUICK *Reference's*

1 & 1/2 cup	335 ml
2 cup	475 ml
3 cup	710 ml
4 cup	1 litre

2 cup = 1 pint   4 cup = 2 pint = 1 quart   4 quart = 1 gallon

1 inch = 2.5 centimetres

8 7 6 5 4 3 2 1 0

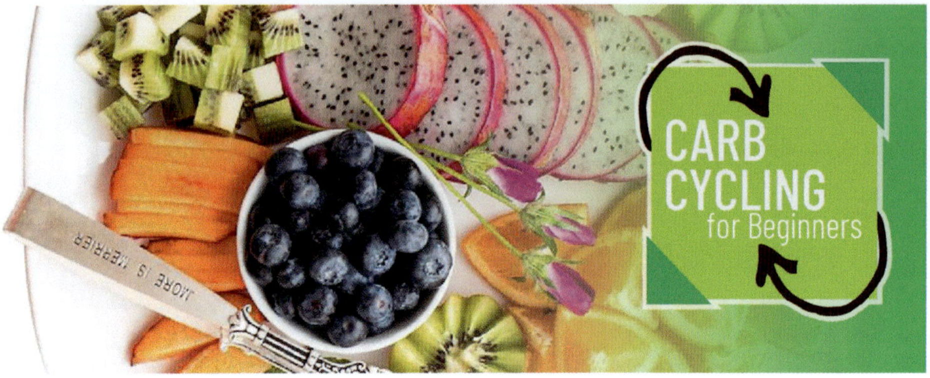

Contact

If you would like to contact me directly or enquire about private coaching, there are a few ways to do so:

www.facebook.com/groups/carbcyclingforbeginners

www.Instagram.com/carbcyclingqueen

+0034 625 497 024

ccforbeginners@hotmail.com

Printed in Great Britain
by Amazon

65470748R00048